Why I Called My Sister Harry

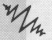

By a recovered stammerer

MICHAEL O'SHEA

Trafford
PUBLISHING

Edited by Nichola Beresford
Cover Designed/Artwork by Graphic Image Ltd.

Order this book online at www.trafford.com
or email orders@trafford.com

Most Trafford titles are also available at major online book retailers.

Printed in the United States of America.

ISBN: 978-1-4251-4164-6 (sc)
ISBN: 978-1-4251-4165-3 (e)

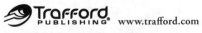 www.trafford.com

North America & international
toll-free: 1 888 232 4444 (USA & Canada)
phone: 250 383 6864 ♦ fax: 812 355 4082

This book is dedicated to people everywhere who are affected by stammering/stuttering and also to those who give so much of themselves in helping to support and empower others to break the silence and become free.

What Has Been Said So Far......

"This is a well written life story providing comprehensive insights into how something like stuttering can consume one's life."

Mark Irwin, Chairman International Stuttering Association

"This book is an important contribution to the cause of helping those who stutter, their families and professionals."

Lee Reeves, Chairman of The National Stuttering Association of America

"Michael O'Shea has given a detailed and revealing account of the evolution and impact of stuttering on his life as well as a deep understanding of his recovery. Nobody has documented the recovery process quite as clearly or as brilliantly. A must read for stutterers, therapists, family and friends."

**John Harrison Author of
"How to Conquer Your Fears of Speaking Before People"
And Founder Member of the
National Stuttering Association of America**

"Without doubt this book should be in every primary and secondary school. In fact it should be anywhere there might be children or young people who stutter"

K Grant. School Principal and Teacher

"I would have no hesitation in recommending this book to my clients."

Trudy Stewert, Senior Speech and Language Therapist

"Being the daughter of a stutterer and a school teacher this book reso-nated with me on many different levels."

T. Maher, Primary School Teacher

"It's all there and it's for everyone; for those who stutter, who live with people who stutter and for those who work with people who stutter. I found the book I would like to see on the big screen."

Anita S Bloom, Vice-Chair,
ELSA (European League of Stuttering Association)

Michael O'Shea has captured not only what it is to live the horrors of stuttering but the immense freedom once it is conquered. No book like this has ever been written. Brutally honest and concisely written, it is a story that people who stutter, friends and family of those who stutter can relate to. One of those books that you can't put down until the end. I can only feel a sense of pride that the programme I found has inspired such a book."

David McGuire Founder of
The McGuire Programme Freedoms Road

Contents

My Road to Recovery

Help Section

Why I call this book my favourite

I met Michael in Dublin. He approached me after a workshop, telling me he was working on a book about stuttering and about his recovery.

Yeah right. I've read many books about stuttering, about how to cure stuttering, about how speech works, even those few with personal stories. So what's new? And this guy didn't stutter at all, so this book would probably be about the "perfect cure", looking for new clients. However, as he was such a nice guy, I gave him the benefit of the doubt and promised to write something and then forgot all about it.

This was my first mistake.

One year later I met Michael again, this time with his wife Monica. I felt ashamed about not writing back, so I tried to avoid them for days.

That was my second mistake.

Then I went to their workshop. Michael spoke about his life having this severe stutter, his battle to speak, physically and psychologically, his love for his wife, work and children, his strength to walk on and make his life a success despite his stutter, and his way to recovery by finding the therapy that was right for him. He told us to trust ourselves, to follow our dreams and to believe that there is a way out once you found the direction that's right for you, no matter what that direction is. What really hit me was that, for the first time, I heard a spouse speak about the impact of being a partner to someone who stutters, but also about the "redundancy" of being a partner to a recovered stutterer who got his speech back. That made my waterfalls burst. And, as they said, it's all in the book. So when Michael asked people to review a draft of the book and take one home, I was like a starving bird and would have fought for a copy if I had to. I walked off with the book under my arm and a poem on my mind. Unfortunately this was the last evening and there was no time to sit and talk to them.

Now that was my third mistake.

I came home and read the book and at 2.50am I switched off the light. This book IS about stuttering and IS about recovery, but it is mainly about life, love, work, family, country life birth and death. As it's so eloquently and vividly written, you can smell the newly har-vested grain, taste the fresh vegetables directly picked from the field, feel the painful punishment from the teacher, see the beautiful but fearful wedding ceremony and imagine the funny sight of Monica with her feet on the dashboard. It's so private, so emotional and so recognisable for many of us who stutter. The book ends with stories from people like you and me, who have "been there, done that" and advice to parents, children and teachers.

It's all there for and it's for everyone; for those who stutter, those who live with people who stutter and for those who work with people who stutter. I found THE book I would like to see on the white screen.

Just one warning before you turn this page. Start early, as you won't be able to stop reading it. As for me, I cant wait to come to Dublin to make up for my triple mistakes.

Michael and Monica, thanks for sharing your lives with us.

A.S.B. (Belgium)

Acknowledgements

This book would not have been possible without a great deal of help from many people. I would like to reiterate my thanks to everyone who took the time to review this book and made invaluable suggestions.

I would like to acknowledge the many people who stammer/ stutter, the many parents and family members, speech professionals, teachers, support groups, stammering/stuttering organisations, and members of the media who were invaluable in helping me to access the information I needed. I have been so inspired by parents who showed strength and character as they pursue the best possible support for their children. I thank you all.

I feel very humbled and privileged that the people who stammer/ stutter had the trust and confidence in me to share their inner most thoughts and feelings regarding stammering / stuttering and that they all gave me permission to publish and relate those thoughts and feelings so that it could be of help to others.

I would like to acknowledge the help and support of the professional speech community. To all who gave advice and knowledge I will be forever grateful. It has taught me that a lot more unites us than divides us.

To the many speech and language therapists, Stammering Association Members, Teaching Association members and the many, many others who have helped; thank you all for your contributions and support.

I would like to acknowledge the many people who helped and supported me in my own recovery from stammering / stuttering. It fills me with pride and passion to see that you all have a new quality of life regarding your speech. You are all fantastic and I will never forget you.

I also wish to thank my loving family. Without your help and support I know this book would not have been written. To my wife Monica for understanding just how much this project meant to me. She cared for me during countless hours of writing and research, and loved me through it all. Thank you for your love and support.

To Nichola Beresford for spending hours advising, drafting and re-drafting this book. Thank you for your wisdom, advice, understanding and friendship in order to make this book a reality. Thank you for being you.

THANKS TO EVERYONE. YOU ARE SPECIAL

Foreword

Michael O`Shea is my name and I was born on July 17th 1955. My parents were overjoyed with their happy and healthy firstborn son. If you are a parent you will know exactly what I mean; that unforgettable feeling on the birth of your child. My childhood, up to the age of four, was perfectly normal; having fun, time and space to explore the usual things that a child of that age achieves. Little did I know that before my fifth birthday a particular incident would change my speaking life, my behaviour and my personality for the next forty years.

Research for this book began in May 2005 and many people have been interviewed; stammerers, speech and language therapists, parents and children. As part of studies over thirty radio interviews were conducted all over Ireland, asking for feedback from the general public regarding their experiences of stammering. The response was overwhelming and some of the true feelings expressed by children and adults who stammer are included in this book. I have endeavoured to choose cross section of people and also those at different stages in their recovery. Stammering/stuttering has no respect for class, race or creed. Thank you to everyone who contributed.

The aim of this book is to help people understand what it is like to stammer. I want to inform everyone how stammering alters your behaviour and your personality. A stammer is individual to the person and because of this uniqueness stammering has baffled some of the best minds in the world of research. They have never come close to finding a cure despite documented evidence on treatment existing back to the 16th century.

The purpose of this book is to make the stammerer, adult or child, aware that they are not alone. Many millions of people stammer in various ways, worldwide. Help and support is available and as a stammerer you don't have to suffer in silence. If you don't have a stammer this book will give you an understanding and insight into this complex problem which has perplexed me for forty years.

I want you to get a full and honest account of each important stage of my life as a stammerer; from where my stammer started to where I am with it today. Many of you who stammer will readily identify with the experiences and emotions I have recorded in these pages.

This book has no scientific jargon, complicated graphs or fancy words. My own experiences have taught me that this can be the wrong approach for many people. I hope it will give you information and knowledge in a very basic and straightforward way. I hope that if you apply it to your own speech it will help you. For parents, friends and teachers I hope it gives you the tools to recognise what is going on in the stammerer's mind.

In a section of this book you will also read personal experiences of many other people who stammer. Personal concerns and worries expressed by Parents, Relatives, Friends of stammerers, People who are working on their own speech, their views and experiences. Many people may find this section of the book the most useful.

The reality is that stammering is now a very serious problem in our society. Bullying in schools and workplaces is only a small part of what a stammerer can go through in their lifetime.

There are many myths surrounding stammering, or stuttering, as it is called in America and Canada. This book will try and expose these myths which are largely based on ignorance.

Stammering is something that we do. It is not something that just happens. Sometimes we feel that we have no control over our speech. Control and a new speaking life can be achieved. You can reach freedom from the shackles of your inner self regarding your speech and your perceptions of yourself as a speaker, but only the stammerer can do this.

The Road to freedom is much easier to navigate with the help and support of other people. Involve other people. I would not be where I am with my speech today without the involvement of people who have no personal interest in stammering; mainly, the general public. Enlisting the support of others is very important if you are to recover and enjoy a better quality of life regarding your speech.

This book gives a detailed insight into my life as a stammerer. In writing this book I have had to be open, honest and expose all of my perceptions, emotions and experiences about how I felt as a stammerer. It would have been pointless to hold back in any way. Going back over my own life as a stammerer has, at times, been a painful journey at other times highly liberating but all in all it has also been one of the most satisfying and fulfilling things that I have ever done.

The research and advice I received have further educated me regarding this mysterious thing we call "Stammering or Stuttering." I have had the good fortune to be in a position to support and encourage more than five hundred people who stammer and I have seen most of them achieve a better quality of life regarding their speech.

I invite you to come on my personal journey and make your own observations of how a behaviour, which is what stammering is, can alter your personality and mindset.

Any behaviour learned by a human being can be un-learned. This book gives you simple, straight forward information and knowledge on how I, with the help and support of some fantastic people, altered my own behaviour and have put myself in a position to be in the world of a fluent speaker.

If you are a stammerer the message is very simple. If Michael O`Shea can achieve this, so can you, for I am just an ordinary person, a carpenter by trade and proud of it. If I can achieve freedom from stammering and a better quality of life so can YOU!

Always remember that you are the real expert on your stammer. No one knows at any moment what your thoughts, emotions, perceptions and sensitivities are. In order to recover you have to change.

Finally before we embark on my journey always remember that, stammering is not the fear of speaking, it is the fear of stammering while you are speaking. It is something we do and only the stammerer can change that. Everything starts and ends with you!

Michael O'Shea

— CHAPTER ONE —

The Trigger

Happy memories of my pre-school years are still very alive in my mind. My family lived outside a city on the south coast of Ireland, in an old gate lodge which was at the edge of a Golf Course. It was an idyllic setting for a young family. There was my mother, Aggie, my father, Pat and my sister Marie, who was two years younger than me.

The golf course, for a small boy in 1950s Ireland, provided a world of adventure. Golf culture was still in its infancy and so sheep were often grazed on the land in order to keep the grass down. The rambling acres of greens were our playground. We knew the golfers and the green keepers and each season brought unique delights. In the spring we'd play with the newborn lambs and when summer finally rolled around, it was time to hunt for tadpoles in the water dykes and run amongst the daisies that appeared over night on the fairways. To this day a waft of freshly cut grass can evoke memories of glorious, playful summers.

The nearest shop was quite a distance from the house, but everyday we would take a shortcut across the golf course to the road that ran along the other side. My mother would buy the day's provisions and off we'd set again for home. I am not quite sure if the lodge had electricity but I know it definitely didn't have a fridge, nothing unusual at that time, and so daily provision trips were necessary. The walk to the shop gave us time to chat to one another and there was also the social side; the people we met there.

My first day at school was in September 1959. It was a catholic convent school. The building itself was quite frightening; big and grey and not very welcoming at all. It was the first time I had ever seen nuns; tall beings draped in sinister black clothing with little faces peering out of penguin like hoods. Of course they weren't all particularly tall, but when you're four years old the world is full of giants. My parents were as nervous as I was. I didn't settle in well on the first day, but I wasn't alone, many of my peers were going through the same torment. I spent three full days in this foreign environment before I even started to adjust. My parents still recall the heartbreaking task of bringing a very distraught little boy to school each morning.

It was only my second week at the convent and I had made up my mind that education was not for me. The golf course was calling and I decided to make a break for it. The day hadn't even started properly as the nun was still at the front door talking to my mother. I knew my only possible escape route was through the door at the back of the room, which opened onto the yard. I had to act fast. The move was swift and off I went. A four year old jail breaker running as fast as his legs could carry him to his only known refuge; his granny's house almost two and half miles away.

We knew my maternal Granny as Nanny Evans. She was a small, petite woman with the character of someone twice her size. Naturally she took the little fugitive in without hesitation but was keen to inform my parents and the school that I was safe. There were no telephones in those days so it took several hours for my whereabouts to be discovered. To this day I don't regret my spirited escape but I realise it must have frightened the life out my poor mother.

I arrived into school the following morning to find nothing had changed. My mind was still set on not being there and once again, as soon as the nun's back was turned, I did as I had done the previous day. This time, however, they knew exactly where to find me. The fatal error in my plan was to run to the same safe house a second time. Of course the nuns wanted me to return to school immediately but my mother and Nanny Evans went against their wishes and gave me the rest of the week off. Together we decided we would make a fresh start the following week. At that time, a mere four years old, my speech was as good as any of my peers. My vocabulary was developing and my progress was normal.

Monday morning rolled around far too quickly and it was time once again to go to school. My mother stayed around until she was sure I wouldn't run away, however, it was only an act on my part. As soon as I knew my mother had gone I bolted once again for the back door, but this time my plans were thwarted. The nun was wise to my route and as I pushed open the door and gasped in the fresh air a large black shadow fell across my path. Another nun was posted outside, ready to pounce if I had made an attempt to escape. They had read the situation correctly and their suspicions were now justified. As I looked up I knew I was in big trouble. This large black figure led me away from the door of my own classroom to another classroom in a building across the playground. The silence between us screamed of foreboding. The other building was the senior girls' school. It was here that my punishment began.

A leather strap came crashing down across my bottom several times. My reaction to this unexpected violence was one of terror and I instantly wet my pants. Having finished with the strap, the nun picked up a cane and cracked it loudly off the large wooden desk. She told me I would get the same again should I ever try to run away from school in the future. Fear and shock had gripped me. Seeing my unfortunate state the senior girls tried to comfort me. My silent fright soon gave way to tears and after the beating I cried uncontrollably all day. I sat uncomfortably in my wet pants until my mother came to collect me. For the following three months I didn't speak. I was very withdrawn and I began to wet the bed regularly. As the weeks went by my parents grew very concerned and called in the local doctor, who assured them there was nothing wrong and that it was 'just a phase'. It would pass.

Eventually I did start to speak again, but my speech wasn't normal. I stumbled over some words and others wouldn't come to me at all. In fact if an adult asked me my own name I would block on it severely. I began to notice that sometimes I couldn't even say my sister's name. If I was excited my speech was worse. Even at this tender age I was aware of the fact that I spoke differently and I withdrew even more. If people visited the house, even relatives with their children, I wouldn't speak until all the adults were out of earshot. I could happily express myself playing games with other children but I was aware of adult reactions to the way I spoke.

I would overhear them saying,

"It must be the shock of the beating in school, he spoke perfectly before then. It will return to normal soon".

Others would kindly say, "He will grow out of it".

If I had a penny for every time I heard that phrase I would be a very rich man. Then the comparisons would begin,

"Jimmy so and so stammered for years, look at him now, perfect!"

What they didn't realise was that Jimmy so and so hadn't 'grown' out of his stammer; he had probably just developed a behaviour pattern to hide it very well.

My sister's name, Marie, was continuing to cause me great problems. She was only two years old then and just starting to speak herself. Already I was developing ways to hide my stammer. I decided to call her Harry. I can't recollect why the name Harry was chosen, but I could say it easily and that solved one problem. It was the beginning of many years of word avoidance and substitution. This proved very useful in difficult situations. I became the master. Everyone, including my parents, assumed it was just a childhood quirk, choosing a pet name for my sister, but I knew it wasn't. I was quickly developing the mentality of a stammerer, a path that would alter my behaviour and personality for years to come.

Although I can identify when, and initially why, I started to stammer, this book is not about blame, institutional abuse or the harshness of corporal punishment in 1950s Ireland. I just want to illustrate the power of seemingly isolated incidents; physical and mental. The psychological impact of the beating I received in school was just the trigger for my stammer. From speaking to other people, in my research for this book, it has become quite clear that my experience in school was not uncommon and many people who stammer have similar stories. The Ireland we live in today is unrecognisable when compared to that time, and hopefully what happened to me in Little Infants would never happen to any child in the current Irish education system. However, this millennium brings its own variety of negative momentous events in the life of an individual. You may be able to identify those moments that pulled the psychological trigger for your stammer.

— CHAPTER TWO —

The New House

In 1960 we moved to our newly built house, just two miles away from the lodge. The house had been erected on my Grandparent's land and Nanny and Granddad were our new next door neighbours. The area had no sophisticated water or sewerage schemes so the house had no running water and was equipped with an outside dry toilet. These were small inconveniences! It was a newly built mansion to us. It was big and spacious compared to the Lodge and my parents made it as cosy as possible. I thought it was great.

My father worked hard all his life. As a construction worker he would often have to travel up to fourteen miles by bicycle for a job. This wasn't unusual at the time and there were many men like him. He had gifted hands and a strong work ethic, which I was fortunate to inherit. My mother was no stranger to work either. She would knit Aran sweaters by hand and pick blackberries in late summer just to make some extra money to make life as comfortable as possible for Harry and me.

Money was scarce for almost everyone in those days, particularly in a small country community like ours, but because everyone was in the same boat no one really noticed. What was lacking in cash was more than made up for in community spirit. We all helped each other out. Our little village was three miles from the nearest city. It was situated in a green valley, surrounded by rolling hills. The magnificent views from the front and back of our house were a sight to behold. We had streams and bogs to play in and the expansive fields to the back often became the imaginary prairies of the Wild West of America. Cowboys and Indians was often the game of choice. There were also plenty of children around in those days and our playtime was driven by overactive imaginations resulting in hours of fun. The days, especially in the summertime, were never long enough.

The village was surrounded by four large farms which provided a great source of local employment. At various times of the year there would be potatoes to pick, vegetables to be thinned or, for me, the summer highlight; the thrashing season. The Ryan family farm lay just one hundred yards from our house. Thrashing involved many, unlike today where the human hand labour has been replaced by the modern Combine Harvester. Thrashing started in the early morning and many men from the village, including my father, were there to lend a hand. It was physical work as the hessian sacks, filled to the brim with corn, oats or barley, were very heavy. There was method in what looked like mayhem, and everyone worked happily in harmony. The women were always on hand with sustenance. Just like the Mrs. Doyle character from the television comedy series, Father Ted, they would arrive with mountains of fresh sandwiches and gallons of tea and lemonade for the workers. When the food appeared everyone stopped working and sat down in the sunshine, enjoying the simple pleasures of a sandwich and a cup of tea with friends and neighbours. Halcyon days indeed!

Water was sourced from the local hand pump that sat on top of a large limestone. Every household in the area got their water supply from here and it was a focal point in the village. Many times a day people could be found filling enamel buckets or other vessels and setting off home with fresh water. Of course the practicality was lost on us as children and we turned the water trough into the great ports of Europe! Our magnificent ships were, in reality, paper boats made from matchboxes, cigarette packages or cleverly folded paper. The field to the front of our house was the place where everyone played hurling and football. Young and old would gather here to emulate the great sporting heroes of the day. My own personal favourites were Eddie Keher and Ollie Walsh, two of the best known Irish hurlers of the time. I would often pretend to be the well known broadcaster and commentator, Michael O'Hehir, and would produce a running commentary during the match. I never stammered during those commentaries but I would only perform them when I was alone. I was often overheard by people on the road or working in the fields. They took great delight in my vivid imagination and impersonation skills; I was totally unaware that they were listening. If someone came into view or arrived onto the Commons the commentary would stop immediately and I reverted to my old speaking self; only talking when asked a question or when I had no alternative but to say something.

My ability to create commentaries reinforced in my mind that there was nothing wrong with me. I could run, play, climb trees, read and add like normal children; in fact in some instances I was even more advanced than most children of my age. The only thing I couldn't seem to do was speak like them. In my own world I could speak perfectly. I didn't even have a problem with those closest to me; parents, grandparents, uncles, aunts and sister, but strangers or new people were my downfall. In an attempt to cover up this problem I would just avoid these situations at all costs.

Giving you snapshots of my childhood is important as I want to stress that it wasn't deprived or unhappy. It was the polar opposite. I have fabulous happy memories of those days. My family, neighbours and friends were the best that any child could ask for. My speech didn't pose huge problems in the early years, mainly because those around me were fantastic and, in their own way, protected me from the outside world. Having moved to our new house I was also sent to the local school. It was a national primary school, which, to my great delight, meant no nuns!

— Chapter Three —

The Boy With a Stammer

For the purposes of this book I have changed the names of my primary school teachers in order to protect the innocent. The School building consisted of three large rooms and just three teachers. Classes were mixed together, with the principle, Mr. Smith, teaching the three oldest groups in one room while Mrs. Flynn taught Infants to First Class in another. The third room was reserved for Miss Jones to teach second and third class. Each room boasted a fireplace where, every day, a fire was lit to provide heating. It didn't produce an even heat and, particularly in the case of the largest room, the fire was totally inadequate.

All three teachers positioned their desks as close to the fire as possible during the winter months. It was so cold that sometimes we were given hot cocoa just to keep us warm. Often a freezing cold day would bring its own joy as we looked forward to the steaming cups of cocoa. The water was heated in a huge stainless steel vessel, known as a 'Burco' boiler

On a few occasions the boiler broke down and we would all eagerly await its repair. As the spring and summer rolled in the teachers' desks would be moved away from the fire and occasionally we would enjoy a treat of a small bottle of milk and a soft current bun.

The building had two cloakrooms and two outside toilets in the school yard. The yard also accommodated a small shed that would provide shelter from the rain, but as it was so small, rainy day breaks were spent inside. Indeed the buildings in the school yard didn't leave much room for a playing area. What there was of it was made of limestone dust with no grass. The teachers weren't interested in teaching us sports even though the local GAA pitch was less than one hundred yards away. We were left to our own devices to run and play. In my school, physical activity was looked on as pointless recreation and not a valuable form of education.

My mother would bring Harry and me to school every morning on the carrier of her bicycle. She would strap our little schoolbags on the front handlebars and balance us like cargo on the back. The school was almost two miles from our home and the bike trip became a daily ritual for my mother, hail, rain or shine. Eventually we would be old enough to walk there on our own. I was around six when we made that first initial walk to school. Everyone walked to school back then. If you were lucky one of the local farmers would pass on their way to the Creamery and we would grab the opportunity to take a lift. We'd sit on the back of the trailer warming our hands on the milk churns as we bobbed along. Sometimes a pothole on the road would jolt the trailer and milk would spill from the churns, splashing onto our clothes. By the end of the school day the stench of stale milk would be left in our wake as we passed. We were never bothered by the fact that we were in danger of ruining our natural aroma when we climbed up onto the back of a farmer's trailer. We would wave to all the other children as we passed them, feeling very pleased with our own regal mode of transport; to us it was the lap of luxury. On the way home from school we often got a lift in a horse and cart. There could be as many as five or six of us on board and it was always a thrill. To this day I fondly remember the gentle movement of the small cart and the earthy, animal smell of the horse.

Mrs. Flynn was my first teacher. She was a nice woman who quickly grasped that I had a problem. Her way of dealing with my stammer was to never ask me a question in class. When she read the roll call in the morning and the other children would vocally confirm their presence, I was told to just put my hand up when my name was called. My mother had informed Mrs. Flynn of my stammer before I started school and at the time there would have been very little information around for teachers regarding pupils with this difficulty. Indeed it doesn't seem to have changed that much today.

I soon realised that every time we were asked to read individually out loud in class, I was passed over. Although I noticed, I didn't say anything, it suited me just fine. Other than reading out loud Mrs. Flynn included me in every other aspect of the school day. Praise was given when it was due and, all in all, I got on very well with her.

On one particular day Mrs. Flynn kept me in at morning break to have a chat. I couldn't have been more than six years old at the time. She gently went through all her questions.

'Did it hurt when I spoke?'

"Did I feel embarrassed when I spoke?"

"Was I afraid that the other pupils would laugh at me?"

Her questions went on but were left unanswered as all I was feeling was confusion. Her kindness and good intentions were not in doubt. All she was looking for was an insight, an insight that at six years old I did not possess. Mrs. Flynn became more and more embarrassed each time I tried to speak and my stammer became worse. Her reaction caused me to notice, for the first time, shame within myself regarding my speech. My young mind wondered why my teacher's face was going red. My little eyes took in the fact that she couldn't look at me when I tried to speak. Was this the reason she would not allow me to speak out loud in class? Harry was asked to read out loud in school, why wasn't I? This new awareness didn't sit easily in my six year old mind.

Two days later Mrs. Flynn kept me in during break again. This time the three teachers were present, as they were having their tea in Miss Jones's room. Although the questions were the same again, it was more alarming as they were being asked by a panel. I was frightened. I didn't really have much contact with Miss Jones or

Mr. Smith up to that point, but I knew they could shout really loud as I would often hear them booming through the thin walls of the classrooms. I was particularly afraid of Mr. Smith as he had a reputation for having a ferocious temper. I struggled as best I could to answer and when I stopped they started to speak amongst themselves as if I wasn't there. They discussed the incident with the nun at the convent in little infants and how they had never, in their careers to date, come across someone so young, with such a severe stammer. They threw around different ideas and means with which they would try and help me speak properly.

I had a stammer but I wasn't deaf! I took it all in. Miss Jones did most of the talking and she came up with a few suggestions like keeping me back after school to practice reading. She also threw in the idea of a teacher reading with me when reading out loud. There were other methods suggested which I can't remember, but all very well meaning I'm sure. At six years old it just added to my confusion and reinforced the notion within me that now there was something wrong with me. Why was I constantly being asked about my speech, why is nobody else kept in a break times to discuss the way they talk? From then on I really began to view my speech in a very negative way. I knew the way I spoke was not acceptable to adults. My friends and classmates didn't seem to have the same reaction at all. They were totally accepting and everything was relaxed, but I could immediately sense negativity from adults. I noticed their discomfort and immediately assumed they were judging me. It was very apparent that this only happened when I opened my mouth to speak. I would ask myself, "is my speech that bad?"

At the tender age of six, I was weaving a label for myself. My self image saw a stammerer first and a person second. Every time an adult reacted negatively to the way I spoke it was just another sign that there was indeed something wrong with me. I was convincing myself of this constantly. I was also getting conflicting messages from the world of giants. My family and teachers were always telling me I would grow out of it before I was twelve and yet when I tried to speak they would look away to hide their embarrassment, which I mistakenly interpreted as disapproval.

I finished out my time with Mrs. Flynn, learning plenty but never, ever being asked to speak in class. It didn't hamper my overall education at this time as I was getting on well in all other areas. I had friends, the teachers were as kind or unkind to me as anyone else but I was acutely aware that my speech was getting worse in some situations.

Returning to school after a long glorious summer break was always tough. I had spent the summer playing in the fields, helping the farmers make cocks of hay, hurling a ball until late into the evening, making camps in the trees and ditches with my good friend Johnny, collecting water at the pump for our neighbours; the activities were endless and the days happy and full of fun. Harry was not quite old enough to partake in the more adventurous games but we involved her where we could. She showed no signs of stammering and it never crossed my mind that she didn't.

When I returned to school that September I moved to a new class and a new teacher, Miss Jones. She had 'teacher' stamped all over; tartan skirt and sensible green cardigans that fitted in nicely with her Hush Puppy shoes. Her hair was always scraped back into a little bun, held in place by a hairnet, and, together with her glasses, gave an air of unquestionable authority. Her severe 'no nonsense' appearance was supported by the presence of a two foot long cane that she would find easy to use when necessary. She was very strict, but, to her credit, very fair, and occasionally her sense of humour would shine through. Miss Jones took her job seriously and in hindsight was an excellent educator. As a teacher she took a personal interest in my progress.

On the first day in her class she welcomed all the new pupils and welcomed back those that were in her class from the previous term. She set the boundaries immediately and wasted no time in laying the ground rules. Within minutes she was calling the roll. The names were called individually in Irish and everyone present would have to answer in the same language.

"Anseo",

(Which in English means present and is pronounced 'on shuh'), rang out as each little pupil responded to their name. When she came to me there was silence. I pushed my hand into the air, as I had been taught to do in Mrs. Flynn's class, and waited for her to glance in my direction and move on to the next name. She didn't move on. Looking out over her glasses, she and I locked eyes.

"Micheal O'Se, you will answer 'anseo' when I call your name", she said.

I tried. I tried and I tried and I thought I would explode. The blocks were so bad on that word. After what seemed like an agonisingly long time, I did it. I got the word out. Miss Jones put her hand on her chin and rubbed her bottom lip with one finger, she then instructed Aidan Cullen, who was on my right hand side and who had answered 'anseo' before me to say 'anseo' with Michael O'Se. Aidan started and I said the word with him;

'Anseo'

It was heard in stereo and it was perfect. From that moment on Aidan was my speaking partner for the rest of my days in national school. When reading out loud, Aidan would have to say his own lines first and then, when it was my turn, he would start and I would join in. It worked. With Aidan I had no problem speaking. Aidan grew up to be a teacher himself. I believed, at the time, that this practice every day in school served me well. I was speaking aloud and I knew then that there was nothing wrong with my speaking voice, but why couldn't I speak on my own?

Miss Jones would often take time out of her own lunch breaks to work with me and reassure me that I was bright and intelligent, often commenting that I would grow out of this 'speech problem'. Those words were common, 'speech problem'. I was hearing the phrase constantly and I was acutely aware of it, particularly the word 'problem'.

The years in Miss Jones's classroom moved on. Sometimes my speech was fine and at other times not so good. Despite it all, I was never skipped over or made to feel inferior. If I was asked a question she would wait patiently and do her best to get me to answer fully, even if it took a while. I often felt that I was holding up the class, but if I was, Miss Jones never let on. She was a great woman with good Christian values and only used her cane when absolutely necessary. The years in Miss Jones's room passed by far too quickly and suddenly I found myself in Mr. Smith's lair!

Standing at just five foot five inch's tall, Mr. Smith was a small man by anyone's standards, but he possessed the temper and aggression worthy of a mythological monster. Despite his lack of height, he had broad shoulders and always wore a suit. Summer and winter the suit was his uniform. In the winter months a grey v-neck jumper would be added for warmth.

His weapon of choice, in those heady days of corporal punishment, was a measuring stick, one meter in length, one and a half inches wide and half an inch thick with a brass feral at both ends. My classmates and I became very well acquainted with his friend, the stick, during our time with Mr. Smith. I still believe that Mr. Smith took personal pleasure in carrying out his varied and imaginative punishments.

He was a Jekyll and Hyde type of character. If another adult, a parent, Parish Priest, or inspector called to the classroom, Mr. Smith's personality would change instantly. He was nice to visitors but the minute they left he would suddenly revert back to his old self. It was very confusing and I didn't understand it, but I knew it was dangerous. Like many teachers, Mr. Smith had his favourites. Life was good if you made it into this elite group. In winter the precious ones were seated at the top of the class, close to the fire and other such privileges were obvious. His teaching methods though, were pretty solid, but his manner put the fear of death in me.

Mr. Smith continued with the same approach to my speech as had Miss Jones. In class when my turn came to speak out loud Aidan would stand up as well and away we would go. Mr. Smith had split us up when we started in his class and so even though we no longer shared a desk, whenever Aidan was in the room he would automatically stand up and recite with me. I am forever indebted to Aidan for those early years. When Aidan was not in school another pupil would be nominated to stand in for him. I always felt this was a burden to them, but I found out many years later that they always felt special if asked to recite with me. They believed that, in their own way, they were helping me get over my stammer. It is only now I realise that my perception was often very different to the reality of any given situation. This misplaced concern and worry just served to confound the predicament.

Mr. Smith would rarely ask me to spontaneously answer a question in class. When my name was called on the Roll Call, if I blocked, he would glance up to see if I was there and move on to the next name. Occasionally I did manage to say 'anseo' immediately, but it soon appeared that it didn't matter to Mr. Smith either way.

One day Mr. Smith did ask me a question. It was early in the school day and he was already in bad humour. It was a cold winter month and the rain was pelting off the windows. I stood up and the words just wouldn't come, the noise from the rain was all that could be heard. I blocked severely. I dropped my head, as I was in the habit of doing when I couldn't get the words out. The sound of the rain was broken by the vicious roar of Mr. Smith shouting,

"Look at me and spit it out."

I looked up immediately, a reflex action to the shock of hearing such a ferocious tone. His eyes were ablaze with anger. I tried again but my state of fear just made it worse. Nothing! Again my head dropped and I started to cry. He shouted even louder this time,

"I said look at me and spit it out!"

The blocks were so severe, he was wasting his time; I couldn't have said a syllable, even if my life depended on it. Mr. Smith was about to explode by now. White with rage he told me to hold out my hand.

He struck me with his measuring stick across my right palm. I instinctively held my stinging palm in my other hand trying to relieve the pain.

"Hold out your other hand", he shouted.

Surely not again, I thought! I put my hand out but pulled back at the point of contact; a total reflex action, my body acting on its own, not wishing to feel any more pain. This just made him angrier. Incensed, he grabbed my left wrist roughly with one hand, drew his other arm back at the shoulder and lashed the measuring stick across, what had momentarily been, my good hand. I cried out with pain. Because he was still holding my wrist with his own hand his accuracy was off and instead of connecting with my palm, the stick came down, full force, across the soft fleshy part of my outstretched hand, just under my thumb. The brass tip of the stick broke the flesh and blood was oozing out of the incision made by the metal. I pressed both of my hands to my stomach trying to ease the pain and then, for the second time in my school years, I wet my pants.

Mr. Smith just turned and walked away. I sat down in my wet seat trying to stop the throbbing pain coming from the end of my arms; they no longer felt like hands. At this stage I was still unaware of the blood seeping out. It was only when break came that I saw I was bleeding. The muscle under my thumb had swollen to twice its original size and was a source of great curiosity for my classmates. A girl gave me a hankie to put over the cut. At lunchtime I confided in Harry about what had happened. I had to, as by then my whole hand had swollen and you could clearly see the width of the measuring stick etched on my skin, a strip of flesh that was now starting to turn a particular shade of dark blue. After lunch the day continued as if nothing had happened, but I knew it had. My right hand had recovered quite well but I was now in agony from the pain in my left hand. I knew if I complained to Mr. Smith that sympathy would not be on the cards, so I put up with the pain until the day was over. Several times I wanted to cry and a voice inside my head was urging me to run home, but I knew the consequences of that, so I just sat there.

As soon as the bell went I did run. I didn't stop until I got home to the safety of my mother. It took quite a while for her to calm me down. I had worked myself into such a state and it had now been festering for hours. My stammer went in to overdrive and I was so bad she had to wait for Harry to get home from school to hear the full story. My mother and Nanny Evans put my hand in cold water to help with the swelling. It was a least another two to three hours before I could, in any way, verbally relate to my mother and grandmother what had happened. Both of them were concerned that my thumb was broken.

When my father came home from work he was horrified. Like my mother, he was a mild mannered, gentle soul, but now he was furious with Mr. Smith. Iodine was administered to the cut and a bandage was placed over it, encompassing the swelling and obliterating most of my hand from view. The next day my mother took me to the Doctor. She examined my thumb, still sporting a clearly visible ruler mark. It wasn't broken but it was quite badly damaged and my inability to tell the doctor what had happened alerted her to the severity of my stammer. The injury to my thumb was suddenly secondary. The Doctor gave us some ointment for it, told me not to go back to school for a week but also spoke to my mother about speech therapy. The doctor said she was going to get in touch with the Health Service regarding that and she also assured my mother that she would be writing to Mr. Smith and the Parish Priest about the incident.

The very next day my father took the morning off work to go and see my assailant. He brought me along with him; a reluctant witness if the truth be told, as I had no wish to see Mr. Smith at all. Dad knocked on the classroom door and you could tell by Mr. Smith's reaction when he opened it, that he was surprised to see us. Very few parents confronted teachers in the 1960s. My father stripped the bandage from my hand and held it up in front of Mr. Smith's face awaiting some explanation. He denied hitting me that hard and said I must have fallen in the playground. Like a great detective my father offered the evidence of the quite visible indentation of the measuring stick. Mr. Smith became quite agitated. They exchanged words and it was made very clear to Mr. Smith that if anything like this ever happened again, to me or to my sister, there would be severe consequences.

When Mr. Smith was asked by my father why he had hit me he didn't have an explanation; when the doctor asked my mother why the teacher had lashed out so viciously she also didn't know. I knew! I knew that when Mr. Smith asked me that question and I knew the answer but couldn't say it quickly and clearly, he got frustrated. The way I spoke made him lose his temper. I knew that my stammer had now caused me an injury. There is still a mark under my thumb to this day.

I returned to school the following Monday with my left hand still in a bandage. Mr. Smith didn't even look in my direction, he just continued as if nothing ever happened. We all noticed that his love of the measuring stick as a means of punishment wasn't as strong after that. He still used it of course, but never again with the side of the stick, only on the flat. Maybe he had received a letter from the doctor or maybe Fr. Dwyer, the local priest had a word in his ear.   Mr. Smith was very inventive when it came to pain and unfortunately the measuring stick was just one weapon in his arsenal. I often wondered if he had read a book on torture ideas or if he was just naturally gifted in sadism. A favourite of his was twisting your hair near the ear and then pulling sharply in an upward motion. This was very painful, but left few visible marks on the victim. He also had a penchant for the ear itself. Perhaps the ears' positioning on the body made it a target. Sitting at a desk, a child's ear is at hand height for the passing teacher; easy to grab. He would catch the earlobe and jerk it in an upward motion. Instinctively, you would move upwards yourself; afraid that the ear would come away in his hand. Very few escaped the wrath of Mr. Smith. During my school years I was pretty much like any child. I misbehaved no more or less than anyone else. I received plenty of punishment fairly and squarely over the years from Mrs. Flynn and Miss Jones but these were always justified. Mr. Smith was in a different league. He took personal satisfaction from delivering pain.

Overall my primary school days were happy ones. Some of my closest friends today were alliances formed at that time. What is regrettable is that there was unwitting constant psychological reinforcement, that my speech was a 'problem'. The kindness of Mrs. Flynn's refusal to draw attention to it, the helpfulness of Miss Jones's interest in it and the cruelty of Mr. Smith's intolerance of it, all just served to endorse the fact that I was a boy with a stammer. The message was clear; the way I spoke was unacceptable; it was bad. I felt very alone about my stammer during those years as it was never discussed with me directly and openly.

The doctor had kept her word and shortly after the thumb incident with Mr. Smith my mother and I began making weekly visits by train to another city to see a speech therapist. This was augmented with a monthly visit to another specialist in Dublin. I was very excited about the first visit to the speech therapist in Kilkenny. At last my speech was going to be fixed forever.

— CHAPTER FOUR —

Sister Monica and the White Coats

My parents were willing to go to any lengths to get help for my stammer but during the 1950s and 1960s there was very little help available. Indeed I was one of the lucky ones to have seen a professional speech therapist at that time. Speech therapists in Ireland were few and far between. Usually they only worked in the bigger cities and, with poor transport and few cars; many never had the chance to go. Ireland wasn't the rich, progressive country that it is today.

I was very excited about my first visit to the speech therapist. I was nine years old and my mother took me by train to the city of Kilkenny, about an hour's journey from home. My excitement evaporated quickly when we finally arrived. The speech therapist was a nun! Needless to remark my last encounter with nuns had left a lasting negative impression. Sister Monica was about to change that view. She was one of the most caring and warm people I ever had the pleasure of meeting.

For the next three years we boarded the train every Wednesday morning to go and see Sister Monica. I would look forward to our visits and they became the highlight of my week. I had to take the day off school and my mother would always make it a day out. The trains were infrequent back then and we would get there at 10am for an appointment with Sister Monica at 2.30pm. The visit would only last an hour but we had to wait then for the train home at around 6pm. The train journey alone was great and it was often followed by picnics on the lawn of Kilkenny Castle or on the riverbank during the summer. In the winter we would stroll around the shops to keep out of the rain. We also had family in the area and sometimes we would visit the relatives. Looking back it was a long day, but my mother never complained. She wanted to do whatever it took to help me with my speech.

The hour with Sister Monica would fly by. She devoted the entire time to practicing with me, reading out loud, voice projection, poetry, speaking in time with a metronome and many other things to try and untangle my tongue. For months I couldn't say her name as I blocked severely on the 'S' and 'M' sounds. At the end of a session my mother would get exercises to work on with me over the week. Practicing at home with my parents and Harry wasn't a problem. I only struggled when other people came in. Instantly something would happen and I would revert back to stammering.

My mother told this to Sister Monica who would take notes and give her opinion. As the months went by I became very comfortable and relaxed in these sessions. I began to speak quite well and eventually I could even say her name. I had made great progress with Sister Monica but she and my mother knew that as soon as I walked out the door I would be back to square one again. To combat this Sister Monica often invited other speech therapists to our meetings. There were at least four new faces that helped me but even though they were all very dedicated, my progress was slow. Indeed the small improvements I was making were not holding up in the outside world. I also noticed that I never saw any other children of my age at the clinic. Of course it never struck me that maybe they came at different times or perhaps were not brought at all. I was convinced that I was the only child in Ireland with this problem. I was alone and unique in the worst possible way. After a while Sister Monica arranged for me to attend a clinic in Dublin. The capital was a three hour journey from home but we made it on the first Thursday of every month for the following two years.

We had to take an early train to Dublin which would arrive into the city at around ten thirty am even though my appointment with the clinic was in the afternoon. My mother and I got to know the capital city very well. Sometimes we'd get on a bus and take a spin to Malahide, Howth, Dalkey or other places just to pass the time. We also got to know all the people who worked on the train. Mr. Kearns, the ticket inspector on the Waterford to Dublin line, always stopped for a chat with my mother and an update on my progress. He would tell me of various people he knew that stammered but 'grew' out of it. I was reassured by his confidence and sometimes he'd give me sixpence to spend on sweets.

Sixpence was substantial enough in those days to buy my mother and me a bag of chips in Dublin. Occasionally Harry came with us and she and I would play in St. Stephen's Green or Herbert Park. My mother always packed sandwiches and a flask for these picnics. The ducks did quite well on our visits as Harry and I took particular pleasure in feeding them the leftovers. I remember those summer visits to Dublin fondly.

The clinic was near St Stephen's Green and, for the first time, I met other children who stammered. There were at least three other boys waiting for appointments any time I was there. The Dublin clinic didn't do anything that differently to Sister Monica, in fact it was the same routine just different faces. I never felt they had the same interest in me that Sister Monica had and so ultimately it wasn't very beneficial at all. As time went on it became boring and monotonous. The exercises I was doing and the advice dispensed to my mother were all too similar to what we were already doing with Sister Monica.

On one occasion I was given various tests by two people in white coats carrying clipboards. I was tested in writing, then I had to put various shapes into their right places on a board, yet another test asked me to spot the difference between two pictures. I may have had a stammer, but I wasn't stupid!

I think the white coats these people were wearing were a little obvious as I was very aware that they were testing me to see if I was the full shilling. Inwardly I found this amusing and I flew through all their examinations with ease.

As I suspected I did very well on all the tests and they informed my mother that I had a very good understanding of everything and that my mental development was above average. I could have told them that; if I could have spoken that is! It made me wonder if the White Coats thought I was just pretending to be a stammerer. Did they think I was just looking for attention and I could turn it on or off at will?

I now realise that these were ridiculous thoughts but they were the real musings of a twelve year old boy. This didn't sit well with me. I was very upset that they first thought I was mentally deficient and then when I passed all the tests they assumed that I was just fooling everyone. This particular forty five minute session completely undid any of the good work that had been achieved in the previous eighteen months. Once again I was confused and bewildered and unwittingly, the adults in my world couldn't explain it.

My mother hadn't been in on the session where I had completed the mental tests. She was only brought in for a briefing at the end. The White Coats spoke to her as if I wasn't there. Invisible again; spoken about but never to, addressed as 'he' or 'him'. In my head I was screaming, "I have a name, I'm sitting here too you know", but I remained silent.

As the White Coats talked my mother became very agitated. She wasn't used to speaking up to people in authority but something gave her great courage that day because I heard her say, quite crossly,

"Surely Michael's school reports and his work with Sister Monica would have told you he was very bright and other than his stammer he is just like any other child."

One of the Coats said, "We were just checking to see if he was normal."

At this my mother blew a gasket and went into overdrive. I was delighted. She quickly and firmly told them that I was perfectly normal and listening to her I was beginning to feel quite confident also. My mother was telling them that I was normal so I must be. She defended my mental ability and was quite magnificent.

The White Coats showed no emotion. They remained composed and detached and said nothing. My mother caught my hand and just as we were about to make our grand exit one of the Coats looked at me and said,

"Michael, say your full name".

Silence. Nothing. I blocked and blocked, with cheeks reddening and saliva running down my face I finally forced it out. The Coats casually noted it on their charts. The White Coats had been right all along. Despite my mother's passion and conviction I wasn't normal. I couldn't even say my own name, Michael bloody O'Shea!

My mother thanked the Coats and we left. The train journey home was very quiet for my mother and me with both of us deep in our thoughts. It was to be my last train journey to Dublin to the speech clinic. The following day we went to Kilkenny to see Sister Monica. My mother explained what had happened in Dublin. Sister Monica was astounded; she said that at no time was 'being normal' anything to do with the issue. Her referral notes, which she showed my mother, just contained her opinion that I was developing all the traits of a confirmed stammerer. There was nothing to suggest that I was mentally challenged in any way.

Sister Monica then turned to me and I will never forget the words she said,

"Michael I want you to realise that you are as normal and as good as any other person. What you have is a speech problem called a stammer. There is nothing wrong with your mind or speaking voice. You will live a happy and successful life. You will learn how to cope with your stammer as you get older. For now there is no cure only control. You are nearly thirteen years of age now. I have gone as far with you as I can go. Practice what you have learned here, you have improved a lot. Whatever you do in life you will be good at it because I can see you have the right attitude".

With that she came closer and gave me a hug and a kiss on the forehead. I could see a tear in her eye and I knew then that this would be the last time I would see Sister Monica.

We said our goodbyes and my mother was visibly upset as they embraced. The train journey home was very quiet for the second day running. It was to be the last time we would journey by train to see Sister Monica. The end of the road had been reached with what the Health Service could offer at that time.

During our lifetime we make contact with many people who have a profound and positive affect on us. Sister Monica was one of those people, I will never forget her.

— CHAPTER FIVE —

The New School

The next school year started in a new building. The new school had been built at the end of the village, nestled between the post office and the shop. It was like stepping into another world. The smell of fresh paint filled my nostrils as my eyes took in the gleaming new tiles and tall glass windows front and rear. New desks and chairs filled the brightly coloured classrooms. There were indoor toilets with hot and cold running water and cloakrooms with numbered hooks in neat straight lines providing a place for each pupil's coat. There were no open fires. In their place modern central heating gave even warmth to every room. Big shiny blackboards adorned the walls of each classroom with perfectly clean blackboard dusters sitting on little ledges just waiting to be used. The teachers had new desks also, with soft comfortable chairs. Outside there was a lawn and tended flowerbeds, while at the rear of the school there were three open sheds for shelter. A concrete play area ran the whole length of the building and, finally the icing on the cake, a dedicated sports field! We had our very own large field in which to play hurling, football, soccer or rugby. It was fantastic.

There were also some new rules. Indoor rubber soled shoes were compulsory to save the new tiles. Each child was requested to bring their indoor shoes in a little duffle bag, usually homemade out of coloured cloth. The duffle bags hung side by side on the numbered hooks in the cloakroom. Because the bags were uniform in size but

unique in colour and fabric, the cloakroom was always a multi coloured feast for the eyes when they were all hung up together. If I
close my eyes I can still see it to this day.

In our old school the window cill level was about four feet from
the floor. Underneath it had dull wooden panelling and you couldn't
see out when you were sitting down in class. This new building was
a revelation. With large low windows the light streamed in and we
had a view. The teachers had a job on their hands to stop us admir-
ing this new found vista. Mr. Smith's fingers must have been sore
from all the ear and hair pulling necessary to stop us looking out. He
had brought his measuring stick with him to the new building but
he didn't seem to use it as much. Maybe the new surroundings had
a beneficial effect on him as well or maybe he felt more exposed by
the windows and was unable to be his true self? I'll never know.

One day a local soccer hero, Alfie Hale, visited the new school. At
the time Alfie was a sales representative for Lyons Tea, a popular Irish
brand, and he was visiting the local schools promoting the product;
handing out branded badges and pens. Although Alfie was very well
known in Soccer circles these were the days of 'The Ban'. It was a
time in Ireland when soccer was frowned upon and Gaelic Games
were King. Now our area was a particular GAA stronghold. There
wasn't even a soccer club at the time, but my uncle Joe brought me to
soccer matches on the sly. I knew who Alfie Hale was as soon as I saw
him getting out of his Lyon's Tea van. When he came into the class
Mr. Smith asked if anyone could name him. I could. I immediately
tried to say it, but nothing came out. I couldn't do it. Eventually one
other boy said his name, but only after several minutes. Again my
stammer had made the difference. I got very used to situations like
this; knowing the answers or wanting to contribute points to a conversation or debate but knowing I wouldn't be able to get the words
out. I just held back. There was no point, I knew I would stammer.

That day during lunch break, Mr. Smith asked to see me. He
couldn't have picked a worse time. We were allowed to play soccer

in school that day because of Alfie Hale's visit, a rare treat indeed, and now I was going to miss it.

When I went into the classroom Mr. Smith was sitting at his desk with Mrs. Flynn and Miss Jones. I was left standing and again it was Miss Jones who seemed to be leading the group. She asked me how I was getting on with the speech therapist. I was asked what school I hoped to go to when I left National School. She inquired if I was being mocked or bullied and other such questions. Over the next few months these little meetings became quite frequent. At first I really struggled to communicate my answers during these sessions but as time went on I became more at ease with the situation. Sometimes I wanted to write the answers down because I blocked so badly. Miss Jones wouldn't hear of it. She insisted I got my message across and all three of them would help me to get my words out. The speech therapist had advised the school to take this approach and I really appreciated their efforts to help. The one thing that still mystified me though, was the fact that they always discussed me amongst themselves as if I wasn't there. I found that quite insensitive and hard to understand. Maybe Mr. Smith believed he had pulled my ears enough over the years to make me deaf!

Looking back I can honestly say that I was never persecuted in school because of my stammer. Even when I had disagreements with my school pals, the way I spoke was never used as a weapon against me. When I was a child it was only in the company of adults that I could see or sense any reaction to the way I spoke. Adults would often comment that I was a very good listener. Looking through their eyes I only saw a stammerer. Whenever I found myself in a situation with adults the first thought in my head was 'how can I avoid speaking'? Later this would progress to situation avoidance as well. It was clear to me that my stammer was taking over my life.

— CHAPTER SIX —

Secondary School

My encounter with the Coats had reinforced in my own mind that I was a stammerer. Regardless of what Sister Monica said, the evidence was there. I was a stammerer, that's just how it was. I had internalised this thought over the years. It was one of my strongest beliefs and it had become very much part of my identity. Every time I blocked, avoided, substituted words, was conscious of my listener, cried myself to sleep or held back when I wanted to speak, I just reconfirmed the belief that I was a stammerer.

When I was growing up there was little knowledge available about stammering, only the myths existed, 'he'll *grow* out of it', being the worst of all. I had no inner resources to deal with the problem. Only one speech therapist, Sister Monica, ever asked me how I felt inside when I stammered. The general approach back then was to look at how you spoke, not why you spoke that way; in other words they should have been looking for the root of the problem, where the trigger was pulled and the stammer started. It took another thirty years before I eventually found a system that enabled me to empower myself to deal with the behaviour that I had internalised and made a large part of my own identity.

The Coats, in their own way, had a positive effect on me. Because of them I was determined to prove to the world that I was normal and prove them wrong. This had a profound effect on my life. I decided that if I was to be accepted I would have to excel in school, sport, work and life in general. I would have to compensate for my speech by proving myself in other ways. My plan revolved around speaking less and letting others know by my actions just how normal I was. This served me well in life but did little to improve my speech. My stammer became progressively worse.

The Vocational School was about one hundred yards from the primary school. It was situated in the centre of the village opposite the Church, which sat in between a Pub and a shop. It had a student catchment area of about five parishes. Most of the pupils came by bus. The bus was free and it was part of a new Government scheme. To qualify for a seat on the bus you had to live a certain distance from the school. This scheme gave many people in Ireland a chance of further education, especially people in outlying rural areas. Of course I didn't need to take the bus as I lived locally.

Most of my classmates in National School moved to the Vocational School for second level education, but a few went to schools in the nearest City and one or two were sent to boarding schools.

The building was modern. It was the late 1960s and, economically, Ireland was experiencing a rising tide and jobs were plentiful. The Government was investing money in education and my school was one of many that benefited. I travelled to and from school on a bicycle; occasionally I walked due to a punctured tyre.

The Vocational School was known locally as 'the Tech'. The first few days were all about settling in. We had to learn where the various class rooms were and get to know the new teachers. Some teachers insisted that we introduced ourselves by standing up in turn, saying our name and where we were from. When it came to my turn I couldn't say a word, I no longer had Aiden Cullen to speak for me. The silence was always deafening. I could feel the embarrassment of the teacher but I never saw it as I always kept my head down. Even if I did manage to get the words out I rarely looked up as I never wanted to witness the reactions. My self esteem as a speaker was at rock bottom but every teacher who found themselves languishing in the painful silence assured me that how I spoke was not a problem. I was comforted by this.

During the breaks we all mingled outside. In those first few days we tended to stay in groups, dictated by the parishes we came from. Gradually those geographical boundaries were broken down and new friendships were born. I was fortunate in that I knew many of the new boys by sight, having played hurling in the surrounding parishes at underage level. I also had a keen interest in athletics and through that discipline I met some of the girls that were at my school.

It wasn't long before I realised how much I missed Aidan Cullen. He could no longer speak for me and I was on my own. When it came to reading out loud I was rarely skipped over. Even though I struggled and it would often take a long time for the words to come out, everyone waited patiently.

Woodwork, metalwork, science and art were my favourite subjects. I found I could really express myself in these areas as they were structured in a practical way; very little talking, just doing. I loved it.

Christy Fewer was the school principal. He was a short man in stature and was soon affectionately christened 'little Christy', everyone loved him. He was a chain smoker who could get through as many as five cigarettes in a forty minute class. There wasn't a smoking ban anywhere in those days. If we were being particularly difficult, Christy's stress levels would rise and require even more nicotine than usual. Sometimes he would spend a whole session lecturing us on the dangers of smoking. He would speak passionately about how it would damage our health and eat up our money. These lectures were delivered through a haze of smoke as Christy puffed away, all the while delivering his speech on the ills of tobacco. I found this absolutely hilarious. From time to time many of the students were found smoking, usually at the back of the Science or Art rooms and would end up before the Principal. Christy's method of dealing with smokers was to hold himself up as an example to all.

"Do you want to end up like me", he'd ask

"I have a constant cough, I'm hoarse every morning and it's all because of this dreadful addiction, do you really want to end up like me?"

The thing was that we all wanted to end up like Christy, not necessarily with the dodgy cough, but as a person. He was well liked and had become a legend in the area. He had a great way about him and an inspiring outlook on life. In class he taught us more than just our lessons. He would often warn us of the 'chancers' we would meet in life. Chancers, according to Christy, were people who would try and con us out of our money. He had a golden rule that he repeated like a mantra,

"If you cannot see it, feel it or smell it, DON'T invest in it".

Many years later these words would ring true. God bless 'Little Christy'.

The practical side of a Vocational School education was fantastic for me. I excelled in the practical subjects and although I encountered problems in the subjects that required speaking, in my own way, I coped with these as well. I made sure I always had my homework done. By having my homework done I would never have to give verbal excuses. The very rare times I couldn't do it, I would make sure to get to the teacher during the breaks. This way it would be a one on one. I knew they would be in a hurry to get to the staffroom and it meant that I didn't have to explain later in class. This was a classic form of avoidance and it worked every time. My coping mechanisms for dealing with my stammer also sharpened my awareness, visualisation and observation skills. I learned how to figure things out quickly. I had to do this so I didn't have to ask the teacher for the answer to a problem. For example, in woodwork class when it came to components in joints I would figure out how to do them quickly by listening carefully and observing more closely what the teacher was doing. In order for the methods to sink in I would use visualisation to put the components together in my mind before I attempted to do it physically. All this effort saved me from having to ask questions. Awareness, observation and visualisation were skills I developed to combat my stammer and they came with me into the world beyond school as well. Ironically, many years later these same skills were my greatest allies in recovering from stammering also.

That first year in the Tech was great. I was accepted and despite my very bad stammer, I wasn't treated any differently. Although I still stammered badly in most situations, when I was with my family and close friends it seemed to be getting better. In school I was always picked first for soccer or basketball games at break times, often ahead of older students from classes above me. On the sports field I regularly took the role of Captain on the hurling or football team. For a young first year student it felt great. For a person with a bad stammer it was bloody marvellous. My life, and how I saw myself, was slowly starting to change.

It was around this time that I started to notice girls. My friends and I became acutely aware of the female of the species and the girls seemed to be more aware of us. It wasn't long before notes passed between boys and girls suggesting who fancied who.

Girls would often approach me and say

"So and so fancies you, do you fancy her?"

I could not understand how any girl could possibly fancy me. Didn't they know I had a stammer? However, I began to notice that most girls seemed to shy away from boys who were loud and aggressive. I came across as shy and introverted. I was the "silent" type in their eyes and it seemed to have a strange appeal. I never had a problem attracting girls in or out of school. The problems only arose when I had to speak.

Christmas rolled around and traditionally there was a party in the school the day we broke up for the festive season. Everyone looked forward to it for weeks. The school had one large room which was divided in two by a folding screen. The screen was pulled back for the party and the room became a makeshift dancehall with cakes, biscuits, and soft drinks as refreshments and a disco. We'd turn up in our best gear and, for some of us, it would be the first time we'd dance with a girl.

At my first Christmas party two friends and I were with three girls. In our own innocent way we had 'scored'. The parties were very well chaperoned by the teachers but we decided to sneak outside. We had previously planned our escape should the opportunity arise. It was a cunning plan. One of us would briefly turn off the lights in the room and amid the confusion we would make our exit, leaving someone else to find the light switch and turn them back on. It worked perfectly and we made our way to the Art room, which with the aid of a screwdriver, we had opened earlier in the evening. Preparation is everything. We had also opened the fire escape door from its latch just in case someone checked and re-locked the main door. The six of us made ourselves comfortable near the fire door exit, should a swift escape prove necessary. Our little oasis didn't last long. In less than three minutes the main door opened.

"Is there anyone in here," said a deep, gruff voice as a hand appeared around the door and fumbled for the light switch.

We took off like a shot out of a gun, kicking open the fire door and climbing over the school boundary wall, dropping down into the Parish Priest's orchard. In our haste we had given no thought whatsoever to the girls. They hadn't been informed of the escape route and were caught by the owner of the deep voice, who turned out to be Mr. O'Callaghan, the Irish teacher. The three girls were furious and didn't speak to us for weeks. Although we weren't caught by the teacher, we had our own troubles to deal with. Our clothes were muddied and dirty from the orchard and this was going to take some explaining to our parents. It wasn't long before a story was worked out. We had gallantly helped a woman change a flat tyre, in the dark on the side of the road. It was a good one and we stuck with it. Over the Christmas break we heard that Mr. O'Callaghan was furious and we returned to school in the New Year with great trepidation.

The first subject of the New Year was Irish! Mr. O'Callaghan strolled ominously through the classroom throwing the evil eye in our direction several times. The girls we had been with were from another class. At the first break the six of us were summoned to the school office. We were divided by gender and the girls were spoken to by two female teachers while we were taken to another room with two male teachers. We were subjected to a lecture on morals, having respect for young girls and the perils of continuing down the wicked road we were on. There was no doubt that if we didn't change our ways we would get some innocent girl into trouble and give the school a bad name. Little did they know that we were so worried about getting caught we didn't even get a bloody kiss.

The six of us were suspended for two days with a severe warning that should anything similar happen again expulsion was on the cards. The girls were given a similar lecture, with one twist; boys like us should be avoided at all costs as we would never amount to anything good!

Interestingly the suspension added dramatically to our reputations amongst the other students. When we returned to school our misdemeanour was quite envied by our peers. We were obviously fun and mischievous. They were right and it wouldn't be the last time any of the three of us would find ourselves being lectured in the school office.

On school evenings I often had to run errands for my mother or Nanny Evans. Nanny's husband, my grandfather, had died some years earlier. We lived on one side of Nanny Evans while my aunt Margaret and her family lived on the other side.

One evening an errand for Nanny Evans took me into the nearest city. My bicycle, as usual, was punctured so I decided to thumb a lift in and come home with my uncle Joe. My mother gave me the usual notes relevant to the messages I was doing. This was one of my best ways to avoid speaking. I'd just hand over a note that explained what I required. This was my general shopping method. If I couldn't point to it, I would write it down and hand the shopkeeper the note. The emergence of the supermarket in Ireland was a huge blessing on my life. I could choose the item, pick it up, pay for it and leave without ever having to say a word.

On this particular evening I was on the main road. I had been hitching for about five minutes without any luck. I was looking out for oncoming vehicles and didn't notice what was coming in the opposite direction. Suddenly a van I recognised came by, I stuck out my thumb, but it kept on going. I wondered why the driver hadn't stopped. My thoughts were broken by a shout from the other side of the road,

"What do you think you are doing?"

It was the Sergeant from the local police station. Aha, so that's why the van hadn't been able to stop.

Approaching me he asked for my name and where I was from. Could I say it? No chance. I blocked severely every time I tried to say Michael. Eventually after a very long time I blurted it out.

"Where are you from?", he said.

Again I blocked so I gave up and just pointed to where I had come from.

"Ballinamona?" The Sergeant said.

"Yes." I managed to say, the fear and the pressure ebbing away.

He proceeded to give me a lecture on the rules of the road. He told me of the dangers of thumbing lifts and that if he caught me doing it again he would look at it very seriously. He also enquired as to whether I had a bike and if it had suitable lights. Then he asked me about my speech. He wanted to know if I'd had any help with it and advised me to take my time and not to rush into speaking.

"Try not to be so nervous when talking" he said.

He went on to say that sometimes when he had to have a word with the "local pups" they would stammer under the pressure. Then he did the strangest thing, he stopped the next vehicle that came along, asked if they were going to the city and told them to give me a spin. As I got in to the van he looked at me with a smile and said warmly,

"Off you go and heed the warning I've given you".

The driver was also from the area and said it was the first time he had seen the Sergeant smile.

As a stammerer, whenever I spoke to anyone in authority, or my perceived authority, such as a guard (policeman), teacher, priest, bank manager, or boss, my speech was at its worst. When faced with one of these people the pressure in my head and chest was immense. The tension would run down the back of my neck and out across my shoulders. Every speaking muscle I had tensed up and refused to work. I had no control over it and I'd wonder every time why this was happening. I'd ask myself the questions over and over; I just wanted to know why.

About twenty years after I had finished secondary school I met Mr. Fewer. We sat in the sunshine and reminisced as two adults about my schooldays and the times I ended up in his office. The Art room incident was still fresh with him and we laughed at the innocence of it all.

A few months before I started this book I bumped into one of the girls involved. Thirty five years had gone by and yet we both laughed about the Art room story also. As we said goodbye her final remark to me was,

"Michael it's fantastic that you cured your stammer, you're like a new man. In school we all used to pity you the way you struggled speaking."

Yes, I had struggled speaking, throughout my years at school and on into life beyond it, although I never really viewed it as a struggle at the time. I spent my energy finding ways of controlling my speech and the various situations I would find myself in. In fact as I rambled on through my teenage years I was beginning to realise that apart from my speech, I was as good as anyone else.

— CHAPTER SEVEN —

The Summer of '69

In the summer of 1969 I took my first proper holiday job with the company that my father worked for. They supplied and fitted shop and bar coolers, blast freezers and chill rooms for supermarkets and factories. Dad had worked there for many years and was part of the team that travelled around the country installing the freezers and chill rooms. My position was in the joinery shop where they made the doors for the chill rooms and other wooden components for the blast freezers. I knew most of the people who worked with my father and one or two of the carpenters and joiners in the section where I was working. The foreman, and my boss, was a very nice man called Pat. He was well respected and ran a happy workforce. I was in my element. I loved learning new skills and this job opened up a whole new world of possibilities. My main duties were keeping the workshop clean and tidy, priming the woodwork, running errands to the shop or builders merchants, making tea and helping out where it was required. I loved it and every day I looked forward to going to work.

Each morning the distinctive smells of different timbers filled the air. Red-deal, pitch pine, Canadian pine, and teak perfumed the atmosphere along with the pungent odours from the glue and paint. The saws, planers and tools of the production floor created the music. The workshop was situated by a river and about one hundred yards away from the Gold Crust Bakery. In the early morning the smell of warm fresh bread accompanied me as I walked down the road to work.

The days in the workshop passed quickly. My tasks were varied and each morning I would make out a list of what the men wanted for their break and lunch. Blaas were popular. These were very soft bread rolls only found in this part of Ireland. Sally luns, brown bread, various meats; the list continued. The shop was about two hundred yards away and was run by a tall bespectacled woman who wore her hair in a tight bun. Mrs. Kearney always reminded me of my former primary school teacher Miss Jones. Mrs. Kearney and I became good friends over that summer and the following summers but it wasn't love at first sight. In the beginning she was a bit wary of me, probably because of the way I spoke, although I rarely said anything. I just handed in my list each morning, she'd fill up a bag with the required items, I'd hand her the money, say "Thank You" and leave. It was only when she didn't have a required item in stock that I would have to speak or point to a substitute. Of course I always struggled when I had to speak, especially if there was another customer there. It was particularly busy around 10am with many of the other surrounding workplaces taking breaks also. Workers from the local corporation, a nearby timber company, local dockers and ESB workers filled the little shop. After a while Mrs. Kearney advised me to drop over the list at around 9 am. She would prepare it and then I would collect it at 9.45am; this plan worked well.

I always looked forward to tea breaks and lunchtimes in the workshop. I was chief cook and bottle washer and I'd listen to the men arguing over sport and politics. They'd tell yarns and jokes and tease me if Mrs. Kearney hadn't put enough butter on the blaas. It was brilliant.

One particular morning I brought my list to the shop at 9am as usual. There was a new girl working behind the counter. Mrs. Kearney introduced Claire, who looked about my age; fourteen. It transpired later that Claire was in fact an older woman and had already hit her sixteenth birthday. She was a very shy girl and so instantly we had something in common. Over the next few days we saw a lot of each other. As well as the morning trips to the shop I would often have to pop back several times throughout the day. It could be to pick up cigarettes for one of the men or to buy extra milk for an afternoon tea break. On one of these occasions Mrs. Kearney wasn't there and I plucked up the courage to ask Claire out.

"I thought you would never ask" she replied.

And so my first summer holiday romance began. We saw see each other every day as we both finished work at half past five, but Claire told her uncle to collect her at 6pm. We also met up every Sunday and we'd go to the pictures or take a bus to the seaside. It was great.

Whenever I had to go to the builders merchants I was given a purchase order with all the items written on it. This was perfect for someone like me. I would just hand over the purchase order and very little verbal communication was required. One day my boss asked if I would help him to clean out his office. We put all the important items into boxes and left them outside. He then instructed me to clean and dump everything else. I was happily working away when suddenly the phone on his desk started to ring. I was instantly paralysed by fear. It was the first time I had found myself on my own with a ringing phone. I believed I was unable to use a phone. Even the sound of a phone ringing could create a horrible feeling in me. Luckily, the ringing stopped and the confusion and powerlessness subsided. It would be many more years before I even attempted to make a phone call. If a call had to be made I would get someone else to do it. I was a confirmed stammerer, therefore the phone was one device to be avoided at all costs.

Claire and I went our separate ways that September. She was returning to boarding school in another part of the country. We had become close and my speech was never an issue with her. Neither was it an issue with the men in the workshop. Another realisation dawned; maybe my stammer would not hold me back as much as I thought. The positive experiences of that first summer job gave me hope that maybe I could have a fulfilling life just like anyone else.

I spent three summers in that workshop and it had a huge impact on me.

I received good advice from those kind men and I greatly admired their character and their skills. They took pride in their work and often repeated the motto

"If you don't do it right, don't do it at all". I soaked it up like a sponge.

I always had a huge interest in sport. As a Kilkenny man, hurling was the main interest as it was for most youngsters in the area. Morning, noon and night I could be found with a hurley in my hand. The first sporting trophy I won was for a 'Round the Houses' bicycle race.

A few of the people in our village were trying to establish a cycling club so they decided to organise a bicycle race for the locals. You didn't even need a proper racing bike to enter, just two wheels of any description. Only one of those entering the under sixteen race had a proper bike and any real road racing experience. A few of the locals acted as road marshals so the traffic wasn't a worry, not that there was much of it about in those days anyway. About twenty of us assembled at the start line. Some had to borrow bikes to partake and there was even one tandem entry. Obviously the guy on the racing bike was considered the favourite with odds on the tandem coming second. The starting flag was a white handkerchief from the pocket of a man who was very prominent in bicycle racing in the city. The official route covered about one and a half miles. There were many sharp corners through the village and plenty of fields to be passed. It was fairly flat, except for two slight inclines. We all lined up, the handkerchief was dropped and we were off.

There were about five casualties at the start due to poorly oiled chains that snapped under the intense pressure or poor navigation. The racing bike was away like a rabbit out of a hole. He was starting to disappear into the distance and soon all we could see was his little backside and all our plans for knobbling him quickly disappeared as well. The race was over four laps of the circuit. The first lap went well; a few more chain failures and several dropped out due to general body failure. At the start of the second lap I went into the lead in our pack of five. I was in third place behind the racing bike and the two lads on the tandem. As we approached one of the inclines I could see that the tandem was in trouble, the chain had come off and was wrapped around the back axle. The tandem was out of the race. As we turned at one corner I decided to make a break for it down the hill. I had gained a few yards by the hurling field, and suddenly I found the racer passing me on the right. He had lapped us. He had only one lap left, the rest of us had two. The racer disappeared around the corner. He was now one lap and one hundred yards in front. First place was gone but second place was up for grabs and there were five of us fighting for it. Without giving a second thought to the racer we ploughed on. Left around another corner, upwards towards the brow of the hill and suddenly it came into sight; the leader, stopped due to gear and chain problems on his fancy racing machine. A fresh feeling surged through the remaining competitors who were mainly on borrowed bikes. The racer was finished and first place was there for the taking. As the racer stood kicking his bike, I took off. Around the next corner I went, but far too fast. I missed the opposite path by inches, but I managed to keep the bike upright. I could hear the crashes with the footpath behind me. Some had made the same mistake but hadn't come out of it as well as I had. I was away with my head down giving my Father's bike all the energy I could muster. As I passed the post office I glanced back and could see the rider behind me. There was about thirty yards separating us. Within a few minutes I had increased the gap to forty yards. I belted along the last lap, carefully navigated the dangerous corner, onto the finishing straight, over the line, home and dry. I had won my first and last cycle race. Only three out of the total entry had finished so we all got a trophy. As far as I know it was the first and last 'Round the Houses' cycle race in the village.

Mr. O'Ceallaigh asked us our names and addresses after he presented us with our trophies, as he wanted to put an article in one of the local papers about the new cycling club. The elation of winning was clouded for a few minutes. Eventually I had to write it down as my blocks were so bad the man could not understand me.

Taking part in the race had been great. I had achieved something honestly and without having to knobble the racer! A few days later I learned that there were politics even in sport. I had developed a love for athletics but that world was not at all pleased about my win at the cycling.

— CHAPTER EIGHT —

The Reality of Having a Stammer

My interest in Athletics started in that first year of secondary school. For the rest of my school life I dedicated a lot of time to training and racing.

When I started running I was average, but after a few months I began to improve greatly. I went on to represent my school over four consecutive years in a county wide Vocational Schools Annual Sports Day. It was a big event on the school calendar, punctuated with good natured rivalry and a day we all looked forward to. I took part in the eight hundred, fifteen hundred and three thousand metre races. As part of my training I would run to and from school on most days. Four evenings a week I would train in the local GAA field under the watchful eye of my school coach, Mr. Walsh, a man called Eddie Hartley and my uncle Joe Evans. Between the three of them they would coach and guide us all through our various disciplines. It was a great time and we enjoyed training and attending racing events throughout the summer. An unusual blend of the smell of freshly cut grass and fish and chip vans filled the air at the weekend and evening race meetings. In the winter months we would take part in cross country races. I wasn't that keen on cross country. The cold, wind, rain, and muck combined didn't make for a great day out. Having to climb over ditches appealed even less and

I could never see the point of some courses, especially when wet. They were quite treacherous and injuries were common. I only ever won about three cross country races and I certainly didn't want to become good at them.

As part of our training we had to eat one or two raw eggs every day. It was good for wind, or so we were told. Many of my peers thought this was revolting, but I believed in it and if it helped my performance I felt it was worth it. It was revolting. I hope modern coaching has moved on since then. As I progressed in track events I began to regularly win or come second and very occasionally third. Mr. Walsh arranged for me to train on a proper track at a private school in the city. The difference between running on a proper track and running around our local hurling field was amazing. My coach at this school was Mr. Leahy. He introduced me to local race meetings in the city and county and Mr. Walsh or Uncle Joe brought me to the events. In the summer I competed in two or three races a week. At one race meeting in Kilkenny, Mr. Walsh introduced me to another coach, Mr. McGrath, who asked if I would like to go to Kilkenny on a few Saturday mornings for training and coaching at St Kieran's College. I was over the moon. I travelled to Kilkenny by train. The coaching was tough and it wasn't long before my performance went up about two or three notches.

When I went into a new environment I very rarely spoke. I always let my ability do the talking for me. Because of this people never got to know me very well and I was often thought of as standoffish or a loner. I wanted to communicate but I always held back because of my speech.

One Saturday Mr. McGrath informed me of a track and field meeting in a nearby town the following Tuesday evening. He wanted me to attend and added that many up and coming young athletes from the surrounding areas would be taking part. It would be a great opportunity to test my progress and he expected me to do well.

I won two of my races at that meeting and came second in the last one. Over the next few weeks my athletics career looked as if it was taking off. I ran at the Iveagh Grounds and Belfield in Dublin. Both places had grass tracks and it was like running on carpet. I had improved my times at both events and people were starting to notice me. My second time at the Iveagh grounds was not to be as successful.

I was running in two races under sixteen fifteen hundred metres and three thousand metres. We were leaving for Dublin early and Mr. Walsh was picking me up at 7.30am. It was going to be a long day so my mother got up early and cooked a great breakfast; sausages, rashers, white pudding, eggs and toast. I scoffed it down with no problem. My family wished me luck and off I went. I was delighted that day that there were two other people in the car. I always hated travelling with just one other person as this put me under intense pressure to speak and I struggled badly in these situations, blocking severely. So far the day was off to a great start.

When we arrived at the grounds I changed my clothes and went through my warm up routine. My first race was the fifteen hundred metres. Coming in to the second last bend I was in second place, right on my opponents shoulder, and on the outside. It was the perfect place for my attack, at the start of the finishing straight. Just as I started to accelerate I got a sudden pain across my stomach. I had no choice but to pull up immediately and sit down. The medics and officials were over immediately but because of my stammer I couldn't tell them what was wrong. I pointed to my stomach. "Is it a cramp?" one of them said I nodded my head. Mr. Walsh came to see if I was alright. After a few minutes the pain subsided and I was fine.

"It must have been something you ate", was the general consensus.

I was afraid to tell them about my mother's fry up just in case they wouldn't let me run in the last race.

The three thousand metre race was another hour away, so I thought I had plenty of time to recover. When the race started I felt fine. I was doing well and I could see my opponent in second place breathing heavily and starting to loose his rhythm. All I had to worry about was the leader. I would make my attack at the end of the back straight. As soon as I started to accelerate again I felt a pain in my stomach; not as sharp this time, but sore all the same. I finished third. I knew I should have won both races. It was definitely the cooked breakfast, but I still neglected to mention it. Mr. Walsh and Mr. McGrath advised me of the dangers of some foods before races. Foods like chips, and burgers. Despite my silence both of them knew that I had obviously eaten something to make me cramp.

Sometimes at the finish of races you would be asked your name. The local club or organisation would want to put the results and placings in the local or national newspapers. Any time I was asked I would never give my own name as I would always block on it. I would say, "Alan Hayes" or "Harry Allen". "Al Hinks" was another one; anything but Michael O'Shea. When the papers came out my parents and friends would point it out and I would always say,

"They must have got the names mixed up".

It is no coincidence that my second son's name is Alan. The only letters in the alphabet that I did not struggle on were A and H, hence my son's name is Alan and I changed my sister's name to Harry.

Two weeks after the Dublin incident I was asked to attend a race meeting in St. Kieran's College in Kilkenny. Again Mr. McGrath said it was important that I attended as there would be a strong field in my events. He also said that a few National Team selectors would be attending.

Two of the most important items in my kit bag were a pen and paper. Before I left home I would write out my name, address, club, date of birth and all relevant details. I would give it in at the registration desks. In return the official would give me my race number and no talking was necessary. Wherever I went I had a pen and paper and that is how I survived. That evening in Kilkenny was no different. As usual I was entering three races. I knew by looking around me that there were a few strange faces in my events, some from as far away as Dublin. In all of my races a few of the competitors were wearing an Ireland singlet, so I knew the competition was tough. That evening I did very well with one second place and two third place awards. I was delighted to have done so well against such a strong entry.

I changed after my last race and I passed out by a table with a group of officials around it. They were preparing to read out a list of athlete's names that they were putting forward for consideration for an athletic scholarship to America. My name was read out just as I went by. I should have been overjoyed by this, but I wasn't. A strange feeling welled up inside and immediately my mind went into overdrive. I knew right away that my promising athletic career was about to come to an abrupt halt. How would I cope if I had to go to America? Who would speak for me in America? How would I explain things in America? I felt sick to my stomach and yet here I was standing on good Kilkenny safe soil waiting for my lift home. America was thousands of miles away and I was, as yet, only being considered, it may never happen, but yet the feeling was horrible. My stammer was holding me in a vice like grip. It controlled me, made me feel inferior and often created unbelievable panic.

Over the next few weeks I slackened off training, made up excuses, missed race meetings and pretty soon it became clear that something was wrong. The coaches asked me over and over again but I was afraid to tell them the reason in case they thought I was letting them down. I was letting them down and I felt guilty about it, but this was my only way out. I couldn't face the possibility of being alone in America with my stammer.

A few weeks later I was playing a soccer match and I went to clear the ball off the goal line. I slid into the goalmouth and damaged my right ankle off the goal post. My prayers had been answered. I was in severe pain, but I didn't have to make up any more excuses about missing athletic training, I had a genuine injury. Many years later I met one of my competing athletes on a speech recovery course. He was a covert stammerer and he had competed for Ireland. We often talked about our time in athletics. One day he mentioned about being put forward for an American Scholarship. Everyone told him it was a fantastic opportunity and how he was lucky to have been considered. Just like I had done, he had also sabotaged his chances. Both of us had only focused on our speech and hadn't realised that we were being considered for our talent, effort and dedication. He was a covert stammerer, I was and overt stammerer, but our mentality regarding our speech was the same.

— CHAPTER NINE —

Examinations

My first state examination was the Group Certificate. It was a big deal. I wish I could say I studied hard but I didn't. I much preferred to go running, or playing hurling and soccer to studying.

The teachers kept reminding us of how important it was to study but I was too pre-occupied with sport and girls at that time to take any notice. The teachers explained that we would have an oral examination in English, Irish and French as part of the overall assessment. The orals would take place a few weeks before the written part of the exams. The first time I heard the word 'Orals', that feeling came upon me again. Immediately I began to panic about how I would cope. I had no one to talk to as no one would understand. I did approach a teacher who told me that everyone had to do the Orals and there was no way out of it. Still, it was only September and it was several months away yet.

Other than this worry school was going well. I enjoyed the practical subjects immensely. The teachers didn't ask me too many questions which suited me. I paid a few visits to Mr. Fewer's office that year, mainly for breaking a few windows while playing ball in the school yard and a few other minor misdemeanours.

The day of the first oral examination arrived and the subject was Irish. We were lined up in alphabetical order according to our surname. The general worry amongst the students revolved around what they would be asked, would they understand the question and would they be able to come up with an answer. I had the added frustration of wondering if I would be able to speak. I had practiced with my teachers. Irish, English, French, it didn't matter; all had been a huge struggle for me speech wise. The French teacher did a session with me on my own. I didn't struggle as much without an audience but it was still painfully slow and I could see how uneasy my speech patterns made the teacher. Faces flushing red, eyes looking away, the usual stuff. This teacher knew me well and was reacting like this, what the hell would the Examiner's reaction be? I had a feeling that they would never have encountered a stammer as severe as mine. At the time I was the only overt stammerer in the school.

My name was called. As I entered the little room my chest was tight and my head was pounding. I could feel the sweat running down my back and my palms were moist and sticky. An unpleasant nausea swept me up. I knew that the teacher would have mentioned my stammer to the Examiner, but that did nothing to calm my nerves. I sat down on the chair in front of this total stranger who asked my name and address. With a huge effort I tried to get the words out. I struggled and struggled, I pushed through on every sound, it was excruciating. I looked up at a very embarrassed face; I read the reaction and instantly knew I wouldn't be in there long. I was asked one shorter question and then I was told it was "Ok" I could leave. I was very relieved but I could also see the relief on the Examiner's face.

The English oral exam went more or less the same way but the French test was slightly different. The French examiner was very nice and spoke in a very calm way, assuring me that I could take as long as I wanted to answer the questions. If there was a word I couldn't say I was advised to write it down. I felt very assured with this Examiner. As usual I struggled but I didn't have to write anything down. I left the room wondering why the other Examiners weren't as good as she had been, she didn't turn red and she never turned away.

During that same year a group of us were asked if we would like to go to a Retreat House in Kilkenny. A few of the other schools in the County would also be attending. It was a weekend retreat, designed to help us develop social skills. We would be taking part in sports, discussing various topics concerning young people and there would be girls from other schools there as well. Retreats were a relatively common phenomenon in Ireland. They usually had a catholic influence organized by priests and lay people. Although they were borne out of a religious ethos, they were designed to be fun. It didn't take much convincing; we signed up and eagerly awaited the day of departure.

We left on Friday morning, arriving just before lunch time. It was like starting school again as initially we all kept to our own groups. The facilitators were young men and women in their 20s. They welcomed us warmly and gave an overview of what the weekend was about. After the welcome address we all had lunch together in the large dining room and afterwards there was a 'get to know you' session. We sat in a large circle and were invited to give our name, home address and school name, loudly and individually to the group. I panicked immediately. Altogether there were about fifty in the circle, ranging in age from fourteen to sixteen and four of the organisers. The task wasn't even going to move around the circle in a pattern, we were to be picked randomly by one of the organisers. I knew I could be called upon at any time and this just added to my distress. I wasn't the only person uncomfortable with this. I thought perhaps they were stammerers as well; they were not.

The pressure was immense, I had to do something fast. I pretended that I felt unwell. This was a familiar routine. I stood up and casually walked from the room without saying a word. Everyone presumed I was heading to the toilet, which I did. In the cool air of the small space I gathered myself. Roughly half the group had spoken already and that had taken about five minutes. I rationalised that if I stayed out for at least ten minutes the session would have started and I would have avoided saying my name. After about ten minutes I went outside the building, by the way getting some fresh air, adding to the authenticity of my 'sick' story. This also bought me a little more time, just to be safe. When I went back in one of the young organisers was waiting for me in the corridor. When he asked if I was 'ok', I just rubbed my stomach and he got the message. He looked genuinely concerned and now I was really beginning to feel sick from the guilt of having to keep up the lie. I was as fit as a fiddle and I felt bad about deceiving him. I couldn't take it any longer, I decided to come clean. I explained that I had a stammer and saying my name out loud in a group was virtually impossible. He was very understanding and that only made me feel worse about lying to him in the first place. I was so ashamed. Great, yet another negative emotion, shame this time, piled up on top of the initial terror of having to say my name to a group and then the guilt of having to lie about it. It was a nasty mix.

We went outside for a short walk. He asked about my family, what sports I liked and if I had any hobbies. I found him easy to talk to even though I did struggle a few times. He said he knew at least four people who stammered. They were all older than me and, indeed, one of them was presently studying Architecture in college. He said that I shouldn't have any worries for the future. He reassured me that I would learn to cope with my speech, but part of that coping would have to involve refraining from lying or making excuses for it. He said that I was an individual and there was a lot more to me than my stammer. This was the first time anyone had spoken to me like this and it felt good.

I agreed to go back in and I promised to do my best to say my name and address at the end of the session. My new friend discreetly explained the situation to the session leader and at the end she stood up and said,

"We have a young man here who stammers, he did not want to say his name at the start as he was embarrassed, but he is going to tell us his name and address now".

I stood up and I felt my chest tighten. Every speaking muscle I had tensed. I paused, took a deep breath and said my name with a small struggle. My address followed with the same approach, a little bit more of a struggle but I got there in the end. The room erupted. They all stood up spontaneously and clapped. I couldn't believe it. Outwardly I was embarrassed, but inside I felt good!

It turned out to be a great weekend. There were debates and discussions on religion, politics, drugs, and sex. We played sport during the day and danced the night away. We met girls and made some new friends; it was super. I left that retreat weekend with a fresh enthusiasm. I believed I would cope with my stammer and I was determined to start believing that I was more than a stammerer. It was just the beginning of a very slow process.

In June of 1971 I completed the Group Certificate Examination. The practical subjects went well and I was confident enough in the others. The results would come out in September, but that was months away – the summer stretched out ahead.

I returned to my summer holiday job in the timber workshop. I slotted in easily as everyone was familiar and I really enjoyed it. This was to be the first summer I was allowed to attend local dances and discos. It took a bit of persuasion but eventually my parents gave in. I looked older than my years so there was never a problem getting in. It was the summer and many of the local parishes held fetes and festivals which lasted for about two weeks. During festival season a big marquee was erected and the dances were held on Friday, Saturday and Sunday nights. These were huge events and most of the big name Show Bands of the time performed. Many a romance started in those marquees and many ended there as well.

The dances were always packed. They were usually preceded by a hurling match which was part of the hurling tournament held in conjunction with the festival. At the discos and dances I rarely had trouble with my speech because of the noise level. During the dance intervals the girls would do most of the talking anyway. I only ran into trouble if we went outside where I was expected to communicate if I was asked my name. I would usually say Alan, Al or Harry. I knew I could say these names easily. Sadly the Show Band era was coming to an end and its demise would bring the festivals down too.

Some of my friends had officially left the Tech after the Group Cert and had found employment. With their new found wealth they purchased motor bikes, mainly Honda fifties, Honda 175s and Yamahas, which were all the rage. On Sunday afternoons we would go to the seaside by bus or get a lift there from one of the lads who had a motor bike. Occasionally we'd swim or play soccer on the beach, but the main reason for the excursion was 'talent spotting'!

On one of these summer visits to Tramore I first laid eyes on Monica Darcy. She had long flowing hair, a twinkle in her eye and a very mischievous personality. She didn't show much interest in me at the time, as she was more intrigued by my friend and his new motorbike.

About two weeks later I bumped into Monica at a dance in that same seaside town. We were both dancing with other people when we spotted each other and before we knew it we were dancing together. We left and took the bus back to the city. I walked her home from the bus stop to her door, which was about a mile away. On the way to her house we chatted easily. She had a great interest in sport, especially soccer and her favourite teams were Waterford United, the local team who were on quite a good run, and Manchester United. That nearly threw a spanner in the works as I support Liverpool but other than her evident poor taste in premiership soccer teams, she was great. She had a bubbly personality and was witty and understanding. My speech didn't seem to have any affect on her at all, there was no negative reaction and we got on really well. On the way home we arranged to meet the following Friday night; our first official date. I left her at the gate, we kissed and I went on my way. I ran about three quarters of a mile to where I started thumbing a lift back home. My feet barely hit the ground I was so happy. On our first proper date we went to see a James Bond movie and had a great night. The relationship was up and running. I didn't realise it at the time, but I had met my soul mate.

— CHAPTER TEN —

Final Year

September rolled around again and I went back to Slieverue Vocational School for the last year. The objective was to pass my Intermediate Examination the following May/June. Life was good. I had actually been looking forward to going back to school. I was running well, had enjoyed the summer with my friends, had passed my Group Cert and I had a new girlfriend. It was a long term relationship, already three weeks old! Life couldn't have been better. Three weeks, by the way, was a record, usually I didn't last beyond a fortnight. This one was different though, maybe because she was a 'townie'.

What amazed me about my Group Cert results was how well I had done in the oral exams. Surprisingly I was marked fairly high. I immediately put this down to pity on the part of the examiner, but I wasn't complaining.

Jobs were plentiful in Ireland in the late sixties and early seventies, particularly in the urban areas. Mr. Fewer and Mr. Walsh, the science teacher, gave presentations on what jobs to go for and taught us interview techniques. Many companies were just starting to do interviews. Up to then getting a job often depended on who you knew. One day a Mr. Healy came to our school to talk about job opportunities with Waterford Crystal who, at that time, was expanding rapidly. They were looking for apprentice glass cutters and blowers. There was great interest in these jobs as Waterford Crystal had a great reputation for paying their workers well and it was considered one of the best jobs in the State at that time. A bundle of application forms were left in the school and were handed out to those interested. Mr. Fewer stressed that we were not to fill out the forms without first consulting our parents.

I discussed it at home and it was agreed that I should at least apply and do the aptitude test. Waterford Crystal was offering a first year apprentice cutter or blower fifteen pounds a week. My father was earning around thirty pounds per week and an apprentice tradesman would only have started on about three pounds per week. Obviously the Waterford Crystal rate was very attractive. Mr. Fewer was surprised at the high number of application forms returned. He would only allow us go for interviews and aptitude tests in groups of four, as otherwise the classes would be nearly empty if we all went together. The tests were simple enough. If you demonstrated the required skill you were called back. Most of the teachers were quite apprehensive about us all going for jobs in Waterford Crystal. They explained the difference in future job opportunities if you were a craftsperson compared to a tradesperson. Obviously with a trade there were more opportunities. Even Nanny Evans used to say "if you have a trade you or your family will never go hungry". Despite the warnings against specialising as a craftsperson, I went ahead with the application.

A letter from Waterford Crystal arrived a week after I had sat the test. I was offered a further three days training and, if I performed well, I would be offered an apprenticeship. Although my parents encouraged me to go for the three day training, they were adamant that I do my Intermediate Certificate before I started working full time; "something to fall back on", as they said.

To be honest I had no intention of furthering my academic education after Inter Cert level. The University of Life was where I was headed, the lure of the money being very strong indeed. Two weeks later I completed the required training, and without even knowing how I had done, I handed the supervisor a prepared letter asking if it would be alright if I did not start the job until I had completed my Intermediate Certificate examination.

I was always very good at planning ahead; having notes or letters written in advance so I could avoid having to speak. One week later I was offered a glass cutting apprenticeship at Waterford Crystal, starting when my Inter Cert examinations were completed in June.

It was already April and the pressure was really on for the last few weeks of classes. A few of my classmates had also been offered places in Waterford Crystal and so being immature and knowing that we had jobs waiting for us, our efforts were somewhat relaxed. The teachers knew it. I, however, did take the examination seriously. I applied myself as best I could. I took it easy on the preparation for the orals. I knew that if I stammered badly and embarrassed the examiners enough I would get a high grade. I was right. Just like the Group Cert, the exact same scenario applied regarding my speech.

Then came the practical exams. I knew I had done well in those and the written exams had also gone well. My time in the 'Tech' was coming to an end. I had really enjoyed my three years there. I had learned a lot and made some great friends that I have to this day. It is also great that I can look back and say that I had the good fortune to meet teachers at that school that left a lasting and profound positive impression on me. The years at the 'Tech' hold a special place in my heart to this day.

— CHAPTER ELEVEN —

The Ideal Job

The world of work beckoned and my first real job started in June 1972. With great enthusiasm I entered the firm of Waterford Crystal, proud to be among twenty new apprentices arriving at the training school. It would only be a short time before being transferred to the real factory. The first and second days went well and I had little difficulty in picking up the assigned tasks. As a stammerer you become very aware of your environment and are always more observant than most. I had an in-built radar to visualise situations before they happened. I was always on my guard so I would be ready to avoid speaking. It was important to avoid being caught in awkward situations.

I watched the Master Cutters around me. They all worked hard for the duration of the day, concentrating on the piece of glass that each one held on the cutting wheel. They were skilful and seemed to have great dedication to their work. This was the perfect job for a stammerer. Solitary and involved with little communication needed. It should have been ideal but my observation and visualisation techniques made me question my decision to be there. Would I be to do this for the rest of my working life? Could I sit at a wheel day after day, taking a glass from one box, cutting it and then placing it in another box? Is this what I really wanted?

At lunchtime two of us were talking to three of the master cutters. They explained that the pay and the working conditions at the plant were among the best in the country but, yes, the work was repetitive and boring. One man said,

"You'll always make a good wage and have a good standard of living, but don't get sucked in; good money is useless if you don't enjoy what you are doing so choose your future career carefully".

I got the impression that all three men in this little group enjoyed very little work satisfaction from what they were doing. Were they trying to tell us something?

That afternoon I watched all the other Master Cutters. They were doing more or less the same thing; some worked with larger pieces but that was about the extent of the variety.

The finished product that these men produced was beautiful and the skill was obvious, but I already knew that this was not for me. During the afternoon I went to the toilet and wrote a note for my supervisor telling him that I would not be returning the following morning. I never went anywhere without my friends, the pen and paper, they were part of my stammering life. The supervisor asked if I would stay until the end of the week. He advised that I give myself some time to think about it and also, at least, I would get a full weeks' wages. I declined.

My mother was furious at my decision and her wrath erupted as she grabbed the sweeping brush and beat me up and down the hall.

"How could you be so stupid" she cried.

It took her about two hours to calm down and even then she couldn't see my reasoning. "The others have stayed, why don't you try it for a few months and maybe you'll change your mind", she cajoled.

It was too late; I had no intention of doing such repetitive work for the rest of my life.

Over the next three months my working life was very varied indeed. Draughtsman, phone engineer (how I ever applied for this post I will never know, why I got it is even more of a mystery), fitter and I even worked for three weeks in a garden centre. Garden Centres were relatively new to Ireland at that time. I had to travel about six miles on my push bike to work each day. That's twelve miles a day round trip. One evening when I was coming home from work a neighbour, who was a building contractor, stopped me and asked if I wanted a month's work helping him to finish off a house he was building just a hundred metres from where I lived. Twelve miles versus one hundred metres; there was no contest. I jumped at the opportunity.

I discovered that I loved working outdoors and the variety of tasks involved in the construction of a house really appealed to me. I stayed with Jimmy until the house was nearly finished, which was about eight weeks.

One day Jimmy asked me to pop over to his own house and pick up a box of 'Lux' from his wife. Lux was a domestic washing powder and he needed it to wash down the timber floors after the plasterers had finished. I knew I could never say the word 'Lux' so when Jimmy's back was turned I ran up to my own house to see if my mother or Nanny Evans had any. I even struggled asking both of them for it, so what hope would I have had with Jimmy's wife? My mother and Nanny Evans had never even heard of Lux, so with my pen and paper I wrote Jimmy's wife a note and off I headed. Even clutching my grubby piece of paper I still paced up and down outside his house before I eventually plucked up the courage to knock on the door. Jimmy's wife appeared and I tried to explain why I was there. The poor woman didn't have a clue what I was looking for, so I was left with no choice but to hand her the note. Instant clarity! As it happened she didn't have any Lux but gave me a box of Tide, a similar product.

Clutching the substitute I made my way back to the site. Of course Jimmy wanted to know why it had taken so long to go two hundred yards to his house and back and he wasn't very impressed with the box of Tide.

"Are you sure you asked for Lux", he questioned.

We got back to work, but I knew Jimmy had his doubts. I'm sure his wife told him she was out of Lux when he went home from work. Once again my stammer had caused me undue stress and time wasting.

Before Jimmy and I parted company he asked if I would be interested in a job with a Building Contractor in Waterford. I jumped at the chance and will always be grateful to Jimmy Coady who gave me my first taste of construction work and arranged my next post for me.

— CHAPTER TWELVE —

The Apprentice

In October 1972 I took a job with P O'Sullivan & Sons Building Contractors, Knockboy, County Waterford. I was just seventeen years old. I was thrown in to work with the carpenters. I was familiar with this world from my holiday jobs in Southern Refrigeration, and Jimmy Coady had also been an excellent carpenter.

In the beginning I worked with a number of different carpenters. I was always very quiet and only spoke when spoken to. I worked diligently and remembered my father's words, "If you have nothing to do, find a brush and never stand around idle, always look busy".

After three weeks I was put with a carpenter called Jimmy Foley from Mooncoin, Co. Kilkenny. Jimmy was small in stature with a fantastic pair of hands and a brilliant mind. He was also very quiet and, strangely, we were a good match. He taught me many of the skills and much of the knowledge that I know. Working with someone like Jimmy was a dream come true for me. He talked very little during the working day and when he did say something, you listened. Having spent a week with him, my boss, Pat O'Sullivan, asked if I would like to serve my time as an apprentice carpenter. I immediately said yes and suspected that Jimmy had put the idea in Mr. O'Sullivan's head. It would mean a drastic cut in wages. As a carpenter's attendant I was earning fifteen pounds and fifty pence for a forty hour week, as an apprentice I had to drop back to three pounds fifty for the same hours. I didn't mind, the sacrifice would be worth it. Kindly, Mr. O'Sullivan backdated my apprenticeship to when I had started working for him. In the five years I was there not a harsh word passed between Mr. O'Sullivan and I. He was always fair.

My parents were delighted and Nanny Evans couldn't have been happier that I was carrying on the family tradition of working with wood. My uncle Paddy was also a great carpenter but he had emigrated to Australia in the mid sixties.

I took my apprenticeship very seriously and was determined to learn as much as I could. I signed up for night classes to complete my Leaving Certificate and throughout the coming years I would do many more night classes to bring me up to speed with other construction techniques. I confided in my uncle Joe very early in my apprenticeship that I would become self employed at the end of my training.

"If that's the case, you had better learn more than carpentry", he said, "You'll need a basic understanding of all the trades concerning construction".

Wise words and I heeded them well. They are as relevant today as they were back then.

Jimmy and I worked every day regardless of the weather. Carpentry is so diverse that we always had inside work when it rained. As part of my apprenticeship I had to do four 'off site' courses in the Technical College in Waterford City. Twenty five apprentice carpenters from all over the country gathered in the lecture room on the first 'off site' course.

The instructor asked us all to introduce ourselves, names and addresses. As stammering embodies the art of holding back, I knew I would be last. The wishing and hoping began. Maybe the fire alarm would sound before he got to me; maybe the instructor would get sick before it was my turn; the same old feelings, hoping to be saved in order to avoid humiliation.

It was getting closer and closer. I could feel the tightness in my chest and the familiar sweat running down my back. My throat suddenly felt like sandpaper. I mentally calculated how many speakers were left. My heart began to pump and I focused on how I was going to say my name. Oh well, they might as well know at the start about my stammer and get it over with. My turn came and I tried to speak. The block was so severe I thought I was going to faint. The room took on a deadly silence and the temperature increased as the heat from the blushing faces permeated the space. Heads dropped in embarrassment and, in shock, the tutor ran from the room to get help as he thought I was having a fit.

He came back with another tutor and I quickly wrote down that I had a stammer and a severe block on my name; I was not having a fit. When the drama was over, the tutor apologised for his reaction, but said he had never come across a severe stammerer before. Could I blame him? Did I blame him? As a stammerer I was used to this kind of situation. Over the next few days all the instructors were made aware of my speech problem as were my classmates. Everyone was very good about it and this certainly took some of the pressure off. I relaxed a little more in class situations. I studied hard and was good at most sports and was accepted as a person and not just Michael O'Shea, the stammerer. It's hard for people to understand but I saw myself at that time as a stammerer first and a person second; it was to be many years before that belief could be turned around.

My years of evening classes and 'off site' time in classroom training produced many similar situations. At the start of each, introductions would have to be dealt with and it didn't get easier; it was just something I learned to live with.

It was difficult to get by on an apprentice's wage. I was taking home three pounds fifty a week and I gave my mother three pounds. This left just fifty pence each week to buy tools and to socialise. In order to boost my disposable income I worked every Saturday with my Uncle Joe who was a building contractor. Joe gave me five pounds for the day which was more than I earned in a week as an apprentice. Sometimes I did nixers in the evening which also gave me extra money and this was quite lucrative.

As my apprenticeship progressed I realised that the more nixers I did the more experience I got. I was working seventy hours a week between everything. I was a good organiser of both time and people, despite my shortcomings verbally. At times it was a struggle to communicate, but it didn't hold me back and the work always progressed well.

Monica was still my girlfriend and we met three times a week. On a Tuesday, money permitting, we would go to the cinema. If we couldn't afford it we would go for a walk. Sunday was always dance night, but again that depended on the financial situation. In those early years of our relationship money was always a little tight. Monica was very understanding when it came to my time. I was attending evening classes and working after hours and she was always supportive. Our relationship blossomed and we started making plans for the future. One of our dreams was to go to Australia for three years. My uncle Paddy had established a large construction firm in Queensland and had guaranteed both of us a job and accommodation. I still had two years left to serve on my apprenticeship and I had to complete that before I went anywhere.

Those two years passed very quickly. Both Monica and I were working and saving hard, but it wasn't long before life conspired to put the thoughts of Australia on the back burner. In 1975 a large slice of my nixer money was spent on a diamond engagement ring. Monica was going to be my soul mate for life. On the 17th of July, my birthday, we got engaged during our lunch break. Life was great and I focussed on the future, stammer or no stammer, I was determined to make our life together a long and happy one.

— Chapter Thirteen —

The Bank Managers

Mortgages were much more difficult to come by in the 1970s. It was particularly difficult if you were just twenty and still had eighteen months left to go on an apprenticeship. Banks and other financial institutions didn't hand out money as easily as they seem to do now. In those days couples didn't go to see the bank manager, just the main breadwinner which was usually the man, therefore this was something I had to do on my own.

Emigration was on the increase and the political leaders were telling everyone to 'tighten their belts' and prepare for the rough times ahead. Interest rates were high and most businesses were starting to feel the pinch. Because of my stammer I didn't approach any of the financial institutions at the start. I wrote to six of them requesting a mortgage of four and half thousand pounds. I intended to build our new home myself on a site we purchased from my uncle Tony. It was next door to my father's parents and my Dad was delighted. My late Grandfather's name was Mick O'Shea and my Dad was thrilled that another Mick O'Shea would reside on Cloone Road. It still means a great deal to him.

All my letters received a response, suggesting I telephone to set up an appointment. I could have saved myself the trouble of the letter! The phone was my enemy so that wasn't going to happen. Monica was learning fast that she was to become my speaking slave. Of course Monica wasn't the only one; my friends, family and colleagues had all been used over the years. I hated having to manipulate people but it was a survival technique, and a huge part of a stammerer's armoury. Monica made all the appointments for the same day in order to get them over with.

I prepared well for the meeting. I made sure I had all the relevant notes written out. I thought about the questions I might be asked and I had written the answers down; the value of the site, a detailed costing of building works, our savings, what was left from the site purchase and our income particulars. The night before the scheduled appointments I didn't sleep a wink. I worried that my speech would be the reason that the banks would turn us down.

The first meeting was at 10am the last at 4pm. I arrived at the first bank, handed in a note saying who I had the appointment with. The manager was very nice, looked at my notes and was very impressed until he came to the part where he saw I was still an apprentice on just twenty eight pounds fifty a week. Even with Monica's wages added, he couldn't see how he could facilitate us. It was against the bank's policy to grant a mortgage to an apprentice. He suggested I call back when I was qualified.

I wanted to tell him about my earning potential, how we had saved and paid for the site in such a short space of time, how I could work three times harder and longer, but, like a vice grip, my stammer wouldn't allow me.

"Thank you", I said, and left.

The next three appointments went the same way. I began to think they were telephoning each other, warning of my imminent arrival, as I got the same spiel from each of them. Maybe all the banks had the same, as they put it, 'lending criteria'. Monica and I met for lunch and she could see from my face that things hadn't gone well. I gave her a rundown of the morning and said that it looked like we would have to wait until I was qualified before going any further. Monica went back to work and I had half an hour to kill before my next 'rejection'. I took out my pen and notepaper and started to write down what I had wanted to say at the end of my four previous appointments. This was the second last meeting of the day. With new notes written down I went in with a positive attitude. The courteous manager looked over everything including the new additions I had prepared in the restaurant. Eventually he looked out over his glasses and said,

"Michael, this is all very well on paper, and I have no doubt you are well capable of achieving what is written here, but you are still an apprentice and the bank will not look at it as permanent employment".

The usual courtesies were exchanged and I left for my last appointment, feeling a little better as at least he said he thought I was 'capable' of what I had written down.

My last appointment was with Mr. Molloy, at the Waterford Savings Bank. He was a very distinguished looking gentleman. As he was the last on my list I entered his office as if I was entering an execution chamber. This was a crucial meeting. It was my last chance and our future depended on it. As usual, internally I was in bits. Heart racing, sweating palms, dry mouth; I had been through it five excruciating times already today, and it was still unpleasant. I nervously handed Mr. Molloy the relevant paperwork. He took his time and read it carefully, some parts he read twice and then said,

"This is very impressive Michael".

Then he asked me a question. I struggled badly when answering but Mr. Molloy didn't flinch.

"I want you to say that again, this time take your time and look at me when you speak", he said kindly.

The second time I was more relaxed and although I struggled it wasn't as bad. After a few exchanges he said,

"Michael I have good news and bad news, which do you want first?"

"The bad news", I struggled out.

"The bad news is because of your earnings and the fact that you are still an apprentice I cannot give you a mortgage, how......"

While he was still speaking I thrust the other piece of paper towards him. He was taken aback as I had interrupted his flow of speech and without looking at what I had given him he continued.

"However, the good news is that in my opinion you should have no problem getting a Council Loan for four and half thousand pounds and when you get approval I will sanction bridging finance so you can start work immediately".

I was in shock and it was written all over my face, had he been a woman I would have jumped up and kissed him, I was so happy. He then looked down at the note and smiled as he said,

"I am in banking a long time Michael and it is very rarely that someone who is only twenty years of age walks in here looking for a mortgage and has a site purchased in advance as well. I made up my mind about you ever before I looked at your last note, and I'm glad I did".

After he explained about the council loan and what I had to do I thanked him and was about to leave when he said,

"Michael, never let your stammer hold you back, there are some great people all over the world who speak just like you, it is nothing to be ashamed of, just take your time and don't rush when you are speaking. By the way how long do you think it will take you to pay off the mortgage?"

"I'll have it paid before I'm thirty", I struggled.

"I'm sure you will Michael", he said, "I'm sure you will".

Monica worked no more then one hundred yards from the bank, I floated over there I was so delighted. Monica cried tears of happiness at the news. That night we went for a long walk, we talked about and planned our future home and we set a date for our wedding; the 30th July 1977. Our new home would be finished by then. I would make sure of that.

Six weeks later I was back in Mr. Molloy's office signing the relevant paper work for the Bridging Finance. Kilkenny County Council had granted us a housing loan of four and a half thousand pounds and we would get a Government Grant of three hundred pounds. We had a total of four thousand eight hundred pounds to spend on our dream home. Mr. Molloy wished me the best of luck and I will never forget all the advice he gave me. If it was not for him I would never have known I was entitled to a Council loan or grant. Plenty of planning and work lay ahead over the next twelve months including something that was sometimes keeping me awake at night.

— CHAPTER FOURTEEN —

Laying Foundations

Work started on our new home in July 1976. We knew that many sacrifices would have to be made over the coming twelve months. We agreed that we would still see each other on Tuesday, Friday and Sunday nights. Evening classes and evening and weekend work for anyone else would have to be cut out as all my spare time and energy would be spent building our own home. My father and I worked every week-end putting in long hours. Sometimes the working day would stretch to an exhausting seventeen or eighteen hours. It was a relentless effort to complete our home in just twelve months of spare time. It wasn't easy but goodwill was abundant and at times Uncle Joe and Tony would help out. We only made two concessions, we didn't work Easter Sunday or Christmas day.

Monica and I had to have a reality check on our finances in January 1977. We had planned a big wedding ceremony with more than one hundred guests. We had already paid a deposit on the wedding reception, car hire, and photographer but when we did the sums that January we realised that we could never save enough money in just seven months to meet the cost. Burdening either of our parents with the expense was out of the question, even though they both offered to. Independence seemed to be our trademark. With that in mind we swallowed our pride and announced that we were having a small family wedding. We were not going into debt for a wedding when finishing our future home was the priority. We also realised that we would need our own transport. We would have to borrow money for that also. That January financial audit was to be a life long lesson. To this day Monica and I sit down in January each year and carry out a 'reality check'. It has been very good to us.

Up to the time that we started building our own home we had been footloose and fancy free. We enjoyed great times, particularly with our very good friends Marie and Jimmy. We went away for camping weekends, trips up and down the country and even a holiday in the Isle of Man. It was the first time any of us had been on a plane. Ten days in the Isle of Man cost us thirty five pounds each for bed, breakfast and an evening meal. The craic was mighty. In the summer months we would go for picnics to the sand hills in Tramore. Monica and Marie would make sandwiches and fill hot flasks of tea. Jimmy had just bought his first car, a Morris Minor. We fondly named her Moggie and she became the fifth member of the group. We'd load her up and head for the coastline where we'd spend the day down on the sand hills playing games. There was innocence in rolling down the giant mounds of sand, enjoying the tea and sandwiches, planning our futures; it was simple stuff but we revelled in it all.

On one occasion we went for a camping weekend to another lovely place in Co. Waterford called Woodstown. There is a great beach at this spot and we swam and sunbathed for hours. When the tide was out we picked cockles and periwinkles and cooked them on a makeshift fire on the beach. We ate them sand and all, as if they were a rare delicacy; gorgeous, I can still taste them even now. Jimmy often had to make two trips to Woodstown. He'd bring us out and then go back for the tent, sleeping bags, food and, of course, Monica and Marie's clothes. Why women brought so many clothes for a long week-end baffled Jimmy and I. Thirty years on and things haven't changed!

On one Bank Holiday week-end the weather turned nasty on the Saturday night. High winds and rain howled around the tent and continued into Sunday. We went to mass in the next village, Dunmore East, and when we came out of the midday service it was still lashing rain. As we travelled back to Woodstown the rain belted off Moggie's windscreen, there was no let up; it was getting worse by the minute. We were starving. We hadn't eaten because we couldn't light the gas stove inside the tent and the wind and rain made it impossible to light it outside. We were hungry with little hope of getting any food. When we got back to the tent the first thing we noticed was that there were a lot of strange footprints in the wet sand right in front of the tent. First reactions were 'we've been robbed'. I opened the zip quickly and was convinced I was seeing things. Inside the tent was a large covered steel cooking dish filled with roast beef, roast spuds and vegetables and a large dish of apple crumble. I thought I was hallucinating from the hunger. All was soon revealed. Marie's parents, Paddy and Alice, had brought them out from Waterford. I still say to this day that they were the nicest roast spuds I have ever eaten. Alice also makes a beautiful apple crumble. We ate the lot as if it was our last supper.

We had many special times like this and I am proud to say we still do to this day. We often look back on those times with very fond memories.

Through out our courtship Monica did much of my speaking for me. I often felt sorry for her, especially in social situations. Where the other girl's partners could order a round of drinks unassisted, Monica would have to accompany me to the bar to order my round. It was the only way. I struggled so badly on the names of the drinks that the barman would not understand what I was saying. I always felt sorry for the barman. I could see his reaction to my speech; I felt for him as, I am sure, he felt for me. Monica's own choice of drink was the worst. Her preferred tipple was Pernod and Lime. She very rarely got it as I could never say it. Inevitably she would ask for it and I would always return with a Vodka. At the bar I would get the first syllable out and the barman would always finish it for me by saying,

"Vodka and White?" I'd nod my head.

Monica was convinced that Pernod and Lime was very exotic and not easily available in the pubs of Waterford. I'd come back with a Vodka and white.

"They had none of that stuff you wanted so I got you this instead", I'd say.

It wasn't long before she stopped asking for it altogether. Vodka and white became her drink. I didn't tell her of this deception until years later. When I eventually did she just laughed. Funnily enough she told me at that time that she always hated Vodka, but she always drank it because she knew how hard it was for me to go to the bar in the first place. During this time if I wanted a pint of Guinness I would simply point at the Guinness tap.

If we were at a large social function where there were a large number of drinks involved in a round I had to raise my game substantially. When it was my turn I'd glance at what everyone was drinking, concentrate hard, memorise it, take a quick detour to the gents and write down the drinks. There was no such thing as asking,

"What would you like to drink?" or even, "Would you like a drink?"

What I saw you drinking at the time was what you got. When I came out of the toilet I would pick the quietest part of the bar, hand in my order, grab a tray, pay the required money and bring back the drinks. With the job done the pressure was off until it was my round again. The energy involved in such a simple task was enormous and it continued for years and years. Inside I was drowning in a sea of helplessness.

Our new home was progressing well. Everything was on schedule and Monica was very busy making all the wedding arrangements. The months flew by. In June we went to Dublin to see the priest who would perform the wedding ceremony and finalise the details of the reception with the Hotel. Monica's father John drove us to Dublin accompanied by her mother Martha. Monica had made all the arrangements and it was the first time that I consciously acknowledged that we had formed a good working relationship, as well as an emotional one. The day went like clockwork. All the arrangements were finalised and now all we had to do was turn up on the day. Monica's mother and father could not have been more helpful and when I look back on it now we would not be where we are today without the great help and support we got from parents on both sides.

On the way home in the car the main topic of conversation was the wedding; the dress, bridesmaid's dresses, wedding cake, flower and all the usual stuff attached to an upcoming wedding celebration. The big day was only six weeks away. As I was concentrating so much on getting the house finished I didn't give the wedding plans much thought as this was Monica's department. When I got home that night that I finally faced up to the fact that one of my worst speaking nightmares was just a mere six weeks away. There was no way of avoiding it. This was one occasion when I could not hand in my trusted note. I visualised the nightmare continuously. I could see the embarrassed faces of Monica, my family, her family, everyone that meant anything to me. They would all be there, looking on with red faces.

The most important day of my life would be haunted by the black shadow of my stammer. I wanted to marry Monica more than anything in the world and so despite my fears I pressed on through. I kept my feelings to myself. The first hurdle would be the wedding vows in the church. They required speaking out loud and that was before any wedding reception speech. Having Monica as my wife was all that really mattered to me and I certainly wasn't going to worry her by letting her know my true feelings about our upcoming wedding day, supposedly the happiest day of our lives!

— CHAPTER FIFTEEN —

Our Wedding Day

During the six weeks leading up to the wedding, my nights were difficult. I'd lie in bed, unable to sleep, with the wedding vow turning over and over in my mind. "I do." Just two simple words. The thoughts of the wedding speech brought the sweat out through me. I could actually avoid the wedding speech without too much difficulty. I could just get the best man, Monica's Brother Bernard, to read something for me out loud, but that didn't sit well with me at all. Ultimately my nature prevailed. I am not that type of person. I knew that this was one time when I would have to overcome myself and my feelings. I knew that if I avoided this I would do it for the rest of my life. In the back of my mind, I always believed that one day I would learn to control this awful stammer that had imprisoned me for so long. Unfortunately I also knew that the breakthrough wouldn't happen before the wedding.

On the eve of the big day both families and many of our guests headed off to Dublin. It was a Bank Holiday week-end and every one intended the wedding celebration to be a short holiday. We married at twelve noon on a beautiful summer's day, July 30th, 1977. I was stunned by Monica's radiant beauty as she and her father approached the altar. In an emotional moment her father gave me her hand and we both knelt down as the wedding ceremony began. I didn't hear one word the priest said. I was so focused on my wedding vows that when the time came for us both to stand up I could feel my shirt sticking to my back. As the perspiration spread and developed a film on my body the priest asked the question, "do you Michael take this woman Monica to be your lawfully wedded wife?" "I do", I whispered. I'd said it without a problem. As the priest turned to Monica relief flooded through me. Words are too inadequate to describe that feeling. Six weeks of endless agonising over this had been for nothing. Of course I was not lamenting that wasted time, I was just ecstatic that I had jumped the hurdle.

I thoroughly enjoyed the rest of the wedding ceremony and taking the photographs afterwards. I smiled easily and happily accepted the lovely words from people, wishing us a happy life together. The pressure was off. Everyone else was doing the talking. As we walked to the wedding car to take us to the reception the gremlins re-appeared. The brief respite was over. My stammer was once again in control, and this time it was raging. The reception was imminent and an entire speech loomed ahead, roughly ninety minutes away. The clock was ticking and I don't even remember the journey from the church to the hotel, I don't even remember talking to anyone when we got there. The only thing I remember prior to the meal was my Mother and Nanny Evans asking if I was okay and Monica reassuring me that everything would be fine. Of course my perception of their attention was that I was obviously tense. They could smell it. Why wouldn't they? I hadn't opened my mouth since I arrived. Now I believed everyone could see it, they all knew how I was feeling; maybe they even felt sorry for me. My paranoia just made the situation worse.

At the wedding meal I didn't eat a thing. This is very unlike me as I love my food. The room was very warm because of the beautiful day outside and air conditioning in Ireland was still a thing of the future in July 1977. I took my coat off but even that didn't help. My shirt was wet against my skin; a clammy, uncomfortable, hot sticky feeling. As the wedding speech drew nearer, the feelings grew worse. Thoughts of how people would react sped through my mind.

Red faces, people playing with their napkins, forks, knives; anything to avert their eyes and hide their embarrassment. I felt that I was going to leave everyone down, especially my beautiful bride. I couldn't avoid it.

The best man Bernard stood up tapped his glass and rattled off his speech. Monica's father stood up and made his speech and my father stood up and responded eloquently. The moment had arrived. I watched as the Best Man rose to his feet once more and even though my fear had blurred my hearing, I knew he had just invited me to say a few words. My legs felt like I had just run a five thousand metre race. As I stood up Monica took hold of my right hand and smiled up at me, encouragingly. I started but it was rough. I struggled through as best I could. My speech was short and I didn't care if people understood or not. The cause of my recent sleepless nights was almost over and suddenly it was. Who would ever understand weeks and months of torture for less than three minutes' speech? The applause broke through but I couldn't bring myself to look up. Despite the loud clapping I didn't want picture of red faces burned on my memory forever. To this day I don't know how anyone reacted facially. Of course I didn't accept the applause as a personal tribute. I believed they were applauding because their embarrassment was over. This is how my thought processes about my speech worked. It's also shows that I had an extremely low self esteem as a speaker, not as a person, BUT as a speaker.

When I sat down it felt like some one had opened a release valve and released the pressure from a boiler. Monica gave me a big smile and squeezed my hand. I felt great relief and really enjoyed the rest of our wedding day. As usual the wedding went on in to the early hours of the morning and the craic was brilliant. The following day we went on our Honeymoon. No expense was spared, ten days to the Isle of Man. We stayed in the best hotel on the island and made beautiful memories we have held dear all our lives.

On the first day of our Honeymoon Monica had to remove the rings from her left hand as it had swollen badly. This was caused by me holding her hand at my side during the wedding speech. I was so tense I was unaware of the strength in my grip. Had the speech lasted a second longer she would have cried out with the pain. When we spoke about it she said,

"If some one had hit you with a wooden plank across the chest the plank would have broken you were so tense".

I was totally unaware that I was squeezing her hand because I was so focused on trying to speak.

We returned from our Honeymoon and settled into our sparsely furnished new home. We had the essentials. Monica had given her mother twenty pounds to mind for us before we went on our Honeymoon, so that on our return we would have something until the next pay day. It was two weeks away. We were never as broke but we had each other and we were a good team.

Monica and I returned to work on the 16th of August the day the world lost one of its finest, performers Elvis Presley. It's strange how it sticks in my mind. I was not an avid fan of the King, but I know I was putting a roof on a house the day he died. The sun was shining and the information filtered through as four of us were working on the roof. We all stopped for about five minutes; it was as if some one we knew well had passed away.

The week before we went on our Honeymoon we purchased our first car; it was a white Renault Four, with plenty of room to carry my tools. We called her Betsy. She had a gear stick in the middle of the dashboard that you pulled like a slot machine handle to change gears. We paid two hundred pounds for her and the insurance cost a further two hundred and fifty pounds. It was a substantial amount of money, but for the work Betsy did over the next few months, it was a bargain and she never gave us an ounce of trouble. A fill of petrol cost three pounds fifty pence and it would last for two weeks. We did have to park Betsy on a hill or push her to start, but other than that she was a flyer. She had an 'air conditioning' hole in the floor which doubled as a water feature in wet weather. Often when it rained Monica would have to assume the child bearing position with her two feet up on the dash board because if we hit a puddle the rubber mat, which was covering the hole, lifted up and the water created a pool on the floor. If we were going out and rain was expected she couldn't wear a dress because of the position she would have to take if we hit a flood. Despite it all we loved that car.

Looking back Monica has often said she spent more time pushing and running after Betsy than she did sitting in her. It wasn't long before we traded her in for a better car. Monica's brother in law, Gerry who is a mechanic, came with us to look at the car we were buying. On the way we got a puncture. Out came the jack to change the wheel but the car was so rusted it went straight through the floor. Now there was a second hole so we covered it with another rubber mat and hoped the car salesman wouldn't examine her too closely. He didn't. The deal was done and we left Betsy behind. About two weeks later Gerry called in to the same garage looking for, "an old banger for his wife to learn to drive in". The salesman said he had nothing but a Renault Four and he wouldn't sell it to his worst enemy as it was so dangerous. It's just as well the NCT tests weren't compulsory in those days or we may never have enjoyed Betsy like we did. The new car had the power and strength to move us forward over the next three years. We had a real key to start her up and Monica never had to put her legs up on the dash when it rained.

— CHAPTER SIXTEEN —

New Beginnings

In October 1977 I successfully finished my Carpentry Apprenticeship. At 5.30pm I said goodbye to my workmates who had helped and guided me over the previous five years. The following day I entered the world of self–employment. Another goal reached.

Monica and I had talked about this on our Honeymoon and we both agreed that we would give it our best shot. I knew I had the skill, determination and work ethic required. I also knew that I had to create my own luck. All that I had going for me at that time was Monica's belief and faith that I could do it, three months work which I had put in place over the previous month, forty five pounds, the tools of my trade and Betsy, complete with a new roof rack to carry supplies; humble beginnings indeed. I knew I would learn the rest by experience. Over the next four years I learned the harsh realities of self employment. When I look back now the old adage 'ignorance is bliss', springs to mind. Back then I thought everyone was fairly straight and honest. The University of Life served up a steep learning curve.

When I started my own business I didn't have a business plan or any of the business support that people have access to now. It was a simple process of just getting a job done, getting paid and moving on to the next one. The business details were quite straightforward but I was worried about how I would communicate with my clients. This doubt was always at the back of my mind. It was a track that played constantly throughout every waking hour; "if only I could speak as well as I could work life would be great".

My speech was at its worst when I had to meet new clients. I always carried a sketch pad and if they needed advice on a project I could draw the answer, rather than verbally explain it. It was a huge relief if the client had a prepared drawing because I could point at various things on the illustration. I spoke to everyone as best as I could and more often than not I got the job. In the beginning this used to surprise me but as a good customer once told me,

"We hired you because you could do the job, how you spoke didn't matter. If we hired you to answer the phone then we may have had a problem".

It certainly would have been a problem! No one will ever truly grasp the level of fear that a telephone produced in me. Even alone in my own home I would not answer the phone. I would travel miles to meet a client rather then make a phone call. Monica, God bless her, did all the phone work in the early days of our business. If she hadn't there is no doubt in my mind that we would have failed hopelessly. The amount of time and energy wasted on running around like a headless chicken where a simple phone call would have sufficed, runs into thousands of hours.

For example one evening I got caught on a job that I wanted to finish so I could get paid. At that time I used to pick Monica up after work each evening at 6pm. At 5pm on that particular day I knew I wouldn't be finished on time. There was a phone where Monica worked and there was a phone in the house where I was working but I couldn't bring myself to make the call. I knew I wouldn't get there before seven thirty and it was a wet, cold, miserable November night. She just had to wait. Needless to remark she was less than pleased when I eventually showed up. I then had to lie and say that the phone house where I was working was out of order. These were the days before mobile phones and text messaging. I felt bad enough as it was and now lying to Monica was confounding my guilt. These feelings were unhealthy but this was how I coped in situations like that and I felt powerless to do anything about it. Just being able to speak into a small piece of plastic would have saved me from so many similar irritating moments.

In that first year of business we held our own. We made enough money to pay the bills, change our car, and carry out more work on the house. I worked relentlessly from seven in the morning until late at night. Monica did all the quotations and invoices when she came home from her own job. She also returned or made any necessary phone calls in the evenings. We were learning the whole time. We always had at least three months work ahead of us, which proved that we were doing something right. We didn't advertise because we wanted to see if the business could stand on its own two feet without resorting to marketing or advertising. This just shows how green we were, when you consider the amount of marketing and advertising that goes into promoting any new business venture today.

The second year went more or less the same as the first. We made a few extra pounds to buy new tools and we purchased our first van; a yellow Toyota Hiace. We bowed to the growing faith in marketing by getting the company name and telephone number on the side of it. "**Michael O'Shea, Carpentry Contractor.**" The van was fantastic. It had room for all the tools and materials and it meant the world to me. Monica had learned to drive and so I didn't have to collect her from work anymore; no more standing around on cold winter nights. Over the next twelve months our customer base expanded. The hours got longer to cope with the workload and any extra money that we made went back in to the business and the house. The business was doing well. Around this time Ireland was heading into an economic recession. People were leaving the country to find employment elsewhere, families were being split up and it was a sad and bad time for many. Businesses suffered as there was little money to spend on luxury items and, for most, it was a case of just keeping your head above the water. Monica worked for a company with a fifty year history in Waterford; it was one of the casualties. She got two months notice that they were closing down. She put some of her small redundancy package into the business which helped to purchase more plant and machinery. Monica's steady income had always been the safety net. It was gone and we had to learn to fly unaided. The success of the business was now crucial.

We were now into our third year and, so far, we had avoided any debt. We were making a decent living, the hours were long but that was the way it had to be. One evening in the summer I came home from work early. Monica had cooked a lovely meal and we were having it in the garden at the rear of the house.

"I have some good news for you", she said.

"What is it?" I responded with a smile.

I was secretly expecting her to say so and so's cheque arrived this morning.

"I'm nearly seven weeks pregnant!" she replied.

To say I was over the moon with delight is putting it mildly. I couldn't wait to tell my parents and Nanny Evans. Our first born was due in February the following year. Life couldn't have been better. Monica was pregnant and the business was doing well. I was also aware that I would soon have extra responsibilities. An extra mouth to feed would require some careful planning.

The rest of the summer flew by and we made enough money for a short holiday, our first since our Honeymoon. Monica was really blooming and she was enjoying her role as 'mother to be'. Over the next few months a lot of work came our way and I employed more tradesmen and sub-contracted out some other work. We were pleased with the way things were going. The work was being done right and we were getting paid on time; both critical to a small business.

Over the Christmas holidays Monica and I discussed names for our first child. I decided it should be her choice as she was doing all the work and I would choose the name of our second child, if we were blessed with one. Monica settled on Aisling if it was a girl and Gary if it was a boy. Now you know by now that the only two letters in the alphabet that I didn't have a problem with were A and H. Aisling was fine, but Gary! Well that was a nightmare. I didn't have the heart to explain to Monica that I would have serious trouble saying GGGGGGary. I'd just have to cope with it as best I could and maybe even pray that we had an Aisling! In a way this illustrates just how unaware Monica was about my stammer. I didn't stammer that much when I was with her because I was so comfortable in her company.

Three weeks before the child was due Monica was admitted to the maternity hospital. She had Toxaemia and the Gynaecologist thought it best to bring her in as it was her first pregnancy. I called in every evening after work and the nurses assured us that everything was okay. I could never ask the nurses or doctors any questions. This frustrated me greatly as I wanted to. I knew from listening to other people that Toxaemia could be very dangerous for both Monica and the baby. Ironically the nurses commented to Monica that she was lucky to have such a quiet and shy husband. If it wasn't for my stammer they would have seen a different side of me and they would have been sick to death of answering all my questions.

Our first child, Gary, was born at five am on the 1st of February 1980. I was overwhelmed by the relief I felt on first seeing him and knowing that Monica was fine. The feelings I experienced when I heard him cry for the first time will never leave me. After the birth Monica was naturally very tired and we agreed that I would tell all the new grandparents and Nanny Evans the good news. As I sat in the car just twenty minutes after the birth the worry started. I thought about having to make a speech at Gary's wedding, parent teacher meetings, birthday parties, ringing the doctor if Monica was away and he was sick. The child was in the world less than one hour and I had just run through his whole life; I had even married him off for God's sake!

This was the all consuming effect that my stammer had on my life. As it happened Gary's wedding speech was at least twenty three years away but this shows how debilitating my mindset and mentality was. I was always focusing on speech related situations that were somewhere in the future and constantly believing that I would disappoint my family when the time came. Instead of enjoying and savouring the moment, the birth of our first son, I was suffering greatly under the weight of my stammer.

On the way to my Parents house I realised that our lives were now changed forever. Two had just become three; I had my very own family.

Everyone was overjoyed at the good news. Naturally, they all inquired about his name. I struggled every time I was asked. Sometimes I would let them figure it out by saying, "it sounds like Harry but with a G".

Monica and Gary arrived home four days later. We took to parenting like ducks to water. Monica was one of the most caring and loving mothers any child could wish for. The house was filled with new sounds and smells and we were learning as we went along. Luckily there was always good advice close at hand from both of our families.

Around this time I got involved with a Company who built unique, once off houses. They offered me the sub contract work on the roofing and carpentry. After careful consideration and checking the Company out I decided to take it on. It involved employing even more tradesmen to cater for the extra workload but it appeared to be a good opportunity. The business was busy and the months were flying by. Gary was nearly eighteen months old and he was thriving. Since he was born I had worked very hard and put in long hours. We decided to take a holiday to recharge the batteries and so we booked our first family holiday for the coming August. In June the Company that I was doing the houses for asked if the Carpentry work could be completed on the six houses before the annual builder's holiday in August. The owners wanted to move in and the Company wanted final payment before the holiday period. We worked seven days a week to get the houses finished, which we did by the middle of July. The Contractors would pay us the remaining monies on the last Friday of July. Our invoice for £4,800.00 was paid in full. We lodged the cheque and paid all our employees and creditors and went on our long awaited family holiday.

When we returned there was a bundle of post in the hallway. As I flicked through it I noticed an envelope from a bank that I did not do business with. I opened it to find a returned cheque with the words "refer to drawer" written across it. The cheque was for four thousand eight hundred pounds. It had bounced all the way back.

This was a substantial amount of money in 1982, especially for a small business. For the first time in my life I really didn't know what to do. When we left to go on holiday we had a balance of £5,050 in the bank and everyone was paid. In just two short weeks my balance had been reduced to just £250 in credit. Anger and worry battled for position and I'm still not sure which emotion was worse. I had every right to be angry and worried. I went for a long walk to figure out what I to do. When I got back I got into the car and went to see a few of the other sub-contractors; block layers, plasterers and plumbers. It was the same story with each of them; their cheques had bounced as well. The Construction Company had issued cheques that July Friday for over one hundred thousand pounds to employees, sub-contractors and suppliers; every one of them had been returned. The Company had folded owing over a quarter of a million pounds in debts. Over the next two days I had to contact our employees and sub-contractors to explain what had happened and that even though I still had other work, I wouldn't have the money to pay their future wages so I would have to leave them go. They all offered to come back and help me get back on my feet again but I felt that if I couldn't pay their wages on a Friday I could not employ them. I was determined to go back to square one and start again. We had done it before, we would do it again and Monica agreed. She backed me one hundred per cent which can't have been easy for her as we had Gary to think about as well. Some of the other sub-contractors got stung for a lot more than we did and lost their businesses entirely. Many had to go back to working for someone else. I was lucky as I didn't have all my eggs in one basket and I had other work to fall back on.

In hindsight one of the main things that saved us from going to the wall was that we didn't have any large bank debts. If that had been the case we would have found it very hard to carry on and make ends meet. Over the next two years we worked as hard as we could to get ourselves back to where we were. Several times I would send the electric bill cheque to the telephone company and vice versa so we could get a week's grace before they were presented for payment. We survived this setback and came out the other side. Sometimes when you are going through hell the only choice is to keep on going! Situations like this just served to make us as a stronger family unit, although that realisation only comes with wisdom and hindsight but at the time it was really hard.

It was during this time that I employed a young man named Jimmy. Over the years he became the brother I never had and I trusted him with everything. He eventually became my business partner and, believe it or not, I never had any problem saying his name. Between the two of us we would drive my business and, eventually, our business forward.

— CHAPTER SEVENTEEN —

Alan and Jimmy

Our second son, Alan, was born on the 19th July 1983 it was a beautiful summer's day and Monica HAD found the last two months of her pregnancy tough going as it was one of the warmest summers on record. Alan had decided to arrive ten days late. The same feelings I experienced at Gary's birth washed over me again when Alan came into the world.

This time round it was my turn to choose the names. If it was a girl I'd picked Aoife and if it was a boy we would call him Alan. One of the main reasons I had decided on Alan was firstly it was a nice name and secondly I could say it easily. I used to play indoor soccer and two of the lads that I played with were called Alan. Whenever I wanted either of them to pass the ball to me I could say their name without stammering. I enjoyed saying Alan. When anyone asked me my children's names I would always say Alan first, hoping 'Gary' would come out easier, but it seldom did. I could only say Gary when I was on my own or talking to Monica or Alan. Gary was delighted that he now had a baby brother I went through the exact same mental procedures about Alan as I had done for Gary; the Wedding Speech, parent teacher meetings, and birthday parties. I even figured out how I could avoid having to make speeches at their weddings.

I figured that the Wedding Ceremony itself would not be a problem; no speaking there so that was fine. Just before the reception I would pretend I was unwell and would go to my room to lay down, this would mean I would miss the Meal and the wedding speeches. When it was all over I would make a miraculous recovery and come back for the dancing. This plan sounded very plausible in my head. I wouldn't be leaving either of them down. As ridiculous as it sounds this was how my mind constantly worked. It all seemed quite reasonable and rational to me. One of my main reasons for planning ahead like this was to protect my family and people I came into contact with. I believed that they would be more embarrassed then I ever would be. I felt I had no control over how I spoke so I just got on with my life as best I could. I had developed a vast armoury of tricks and avoidance mechanisms which got me through the speaking world.

I firmly believe that we can learn as much from our failures as we do from our successes. We all make mistakes or have a run of bad luck but we can learn from it. Sometimes it is even necessary to make the same mistake twice in order to learn the lesson. The most important thing that I learned from my experience with the Housing Contractor was never to trust anyone as far as money was concerned. The wise words of my old school principal, Little Christie, rang loudly in my ears,

"There are people out there who are only too happy to relieve you of your hard earned money".

I also found out that banks do not listen to hard luck stories. I had to make sure that something like this would never happen again. The setback hurt us financially but it did not break our spirit. I worked harder than ever, with even more determination than before. Within a few weeks I needed help with the work I was doing because we were just starting to get back on our feet and I could not pay a qualified tradesman. I decided I would take on an apprentice. My sister Marie's husband Frank was working in the Construction Business at this time and he told me about a young man called Jimmy Murphy. He was a second year apprentice carpenter and was being laid off the following Friday. He asked if I could give him a few weeks work.

The next night Jimmy called over and he came across as a nice, polite young man. We talked about his past training. He didn't outwardly react that much to my stammering, in fact he seemed fairly relaxed about it. We both agreed that he would come and work for me on a trial basis for three months and if it worked out I would keep him on to finish out his apprenticeship. To say it was one of my best business decisions ever would be an understatement.

Jimmy became one of the best assets the business had and he is one of the main reasons our business is where it is today. If he had known the financial predicament I was in at the time he may not have accepted the job. Jimmy started on sixty pounds per week. Monica was getting the same amount to keep the two of us and two young children. We had to do this for nearly two years until we got back on track but we didn't let anyone know the position we were in. We made sure that the children never suffered. Santa still came at Christmas, the birthday parties were held and there was always food on the table. They were happy and blissfully unaware of our financial struggles. We kept Jimmy on when he completed his apprenticeship. He was a dedicated and committed worker and we had formed a good working relationship. Over the next three years we worked long hours. I didn't take every job I was offered because I didn't want a large workforce. I had learned my lesson in the past. A small, tight, well functioning and profitable business is what we wanted. It made no sense to me boasting that you had fifteen or twenty people employed if you weren't profitable. Many people fell in to that trap around this time, and as a result businesses failed.

The Tax regime that the Irish Government had in place back then was severe. We were told it was there to combat the recession Ireland was experiencing. Jimmy was working long hours and he was being fleeced by the tax system. I was very aware of this and felt it was very unfair on him. I discussed it with Monica and we decided that I should offer Jimmy a partnership in the business. We had a long chat and he accepted.

We purchased a new van and the company logo was changed to **O`Shea & Murphy Building and Carpentry Contractors.** We are still together today and the business is stronger than ever. We've had our ups and downs but good Business Partnerships are like good marriages, you have to work at it and learn to be flexible but never lose sight of the important things that really matter.

The two boys were growing up fast. Gary would be starting school soon and Alan was hot on his heels. Parent teacher meetings and other social interaction that is all part of being a good parent were just around the corner. I knew I had to get help regarding my speech. I was so desperate I would try anything.

— CHAPTER EIGHTEEN —

Therapy, Faith-Healers and Strange Characters

I had a brief encounter with speech therapy when I was fourteen. It didn't last long and seemed to have little effect and, at the time, was the only recognised help available. By the age of thirty I desired nothing more than to get help with my speech. I wanted the ability to hold a simple conversation, to book a holiday, order a taxi over the phone, chat easily with my children's friends; things that people do daily but take so much for granted. I wasn't interested in becoming a TV or radio broadcaster or even a great orator; I just wanted to speak normally. I made up my mind to try anything and everything to find an answer.

Shortly after Gary started school I began my research in earnest. At that time all I could find were books written by people involved in speech therapy. I found the texts difficult to understand and, even though I tried my best to carry out the instructions, they had little effect. I tried to talk on the phone, with the instructions written out in front of me, but when I started to speak it was struggle after struggle to get the words out. Reading books about stammering was proving fruitless. I needed some outside help. Maybe another stab with an actual speech therapist might work. I convinced myself that at fourteen I was too immature to understand the method. My first port of call was the local Health Service; was there a speech therapist available? This was a dead end. There was no help for adults who stammered!

With one door closed I moved onto hypnosis. I went to a hypnotic show hosted by a well known hypnotist and volunteered immediately when he asked for participants from the audience. Nine people ended up on the stage. The hypnotist asked each of us our names and where we came from. He came to me; I couldn't say a word. The microphone was in front of my mouth and I blocked severely. It was an uneasy moment for both of us. His embarrassment was palpable. A dreadful silence hung in the air and you could see he had never encountered someone like me live on stage before. Silence is not good in a live show! He recovered as best he could with a,

"Maybe – maybe we can help you, just relax. I'll come back to you".

He swiftly moved on to the next person. When he started to hypnotise us I was as relaxed as possible because I really wanted it to work. We knew from the start that he would only keep six or seven of the initial volunteers for the main show. There are no prizes for guessing who was asked to leave the stage first. Two others were eliminated soon after me and the show began. I went to the back of the theatre and watched. That night I waited outside the stage door to meet the hypnotist alone. I had prepared a note and as he left I handed it to him. It said,

"I have tried many things to try and help my speech. I stammer badly is there any way you can help me".

He was very understanding and we chatted for a few minutes. He was honest enough to admit that, in his opinion, all he could do was help me to relax a little more about my speech. We tried. He took my money and I relaxed, but my speech didn't improve. It had cost half my week's wages. I went on to try two very famous hypnotists during this time and although I always paid a great deal of money for the experience, it never worked. It was time to move on.

Faith Healers, Seventh Sons of Seventh Sons, mystics; I approached them all with blind faith and hope that I would have a breakthrough. One woman was sure she could help. She called herself a mystic. When I arrived at her place of work I was handed a white robe to put on. Once dressed, I was taken to another room that had a large leather couch. Soft music played in the background and the space was illuminated by six small candles which also scented the air. Dressed in my long robe I was laid out on the couch. As I lay there soaking up this rather strange but very relaxing atmosphere, the woman, who was also wearing flowing robes, waved large palm branches over me while chanting,

"Leave stammer, leave Michael's body."

She continuously recited this order in a low voice for about thirty minutes. The chanting got a little irritating, but overall it was very pleasant and I did relax. The session finished, I paid my money, but despite her pleading the stammer hadn't left. I was still a stammerer but I was now a stammerer with a great ability to relax!

Whenever I attempted to get help I did it quietly. As far as I was concerned it was my problem and I alone had to deal with it. I generally excluded Monica from my efforts. When I went to Building Exhibitions abroad I would try and find out if there was anyone there who could help. I would have to make extensive arrangements by post beforehand as these were the days before e-mail. I met some very knowledgeable people who had extensive information on the theory of stammering, but theory was of little use to me. I soon realised that I needed to meet someone who had improved their own speech or, better still, someone who had conquered the problem entirely, if such a person existed.

Around this time Monica heard two men who were helping people recover from stammering being interviewed on a radio show. They had brought along two people they were helping at the time. Monica took down the details and I wrote to them immediately.

Within two weeks I was on their course. It started on a Friday evening and finished on Sunday evening. It cost the price of a very large fridge at the time, and was held in an old farm house, way out in the country, and miles from civilisation. The two men who had been interviewed on the radio were the course leaders. They also stammered but had learned to speak reasonably well. They had developed a new technique and had been practicing it with relative success for six months. We were there to learn this technique which they called 'the technique' over the weekend.

There were ten of us on the course plus the two Instructors, making a fine group of twelve. Unfortunately the farmhouse was not equipped for such a large weekending party. In fact the farmhouse was barely fit for habitation by two people let alone twelve. There was a distinct musty smell in the air, every room was damp and there was no hot water. There were only four bedrooms and just six beds between them. Initially I wondered if I was on the right course at all! Everyone was asked to bring a sleeping bag, which was just as well as the few beds that were there were quite damp. I decided to pitch my sleeping bag on the floor, much more comfortable than a soggy mattress. The only heating in the house was a well stocked log fire in the living room which reminded me of my days in primary school; all the other areas of the house were freezing.

It was a wet and windy Friday night and I didn't arrive at the house until around eight o'clock because it was so difficult to find, but I wasn't the last. Six others had arrived before me, all Irish, but from different counties. It was the first time I had ever met a woman who stammered and when everyone arrived there were actually three women on that course.

The introduction started at nine thirty and went on until half past midnight. On Saturday and Sunday we got to experience and practice 'the technique'. It was quite simple; just speak while moving your head up and down! To this day a little nodding dog on the back window of a car reminds me instantly of the technique.

The technique actually worked if you were prepared to use it. On Saturday we went shopping to the nearest town to practice asking for items using the technique. I found it very helpful and it was the first time in my life that I could say a sentence or hold a conversation with someone without stammering. Of course I now spoke relatively well but l looked like I had a strange tic; although the nodding didn't matter if you were on the phone. Everyone on the course improved over the two days, some more than others. It was the first time that I had ever spoken in a group to other people who stammered. The best part for me was that I could talk to other people who came from the same place as I did regarding their speech. I loved that feeling of being with other people like me, people who understood and I wished the course could have lasted a week.

On the way home on Sunday evening I stopped at a restaurant and ordered a meal. I didn't point at the menu once, it was marvellous. My confidence was soaring. I was bold enough to pick up two hitch hikers who were travelling about twenty miles. We had a great conversation; they didn't get a word in edgeways. It was a little difficult to drive, nod your head up and down and talk all at the same time, but this was a small thing to overcome. I refused to be silenced; I felt on top of the world. Arriving home I was eager to see Monica and to fill her in about everything. I told her about the schedule, the house, and the people, where they came from; no detail was spared. She couldn't believe it. It was the first time she had heard me speak without stammering, although she did find the head nodding amusing at times. I didn't care. Now I could communicate reasonably well and that was all that mattered.

Over the next two weeks I continued to nod but without the initial enthusiasm when just emerging from the course, I slipped back a little. The course provided back up in the form of four phone calls a week to the two instructors, but only for the first fortnight. They held two refresher courses over the next four months and then one of them went to England to carry out more research on the technique.

When he returned, three months later, the two of them decided to hold an Annual General Meeting. They had chosen a hotel in Dublin and they invited over eighty people who had previously attended their courses. The object of the A.G.M was to inform us of yet another 'new' approach to stammering and also to practice the original technique.

Monica came with me. I was really looking forward to meeting those who were attending as I always found it helpful just being in the company of other people who stammered. I don't know why, but just talking about our common problems seemed to help my own speech greatly.

The meeting started and the new approach was explained. Basically we were to advertise ourselves as Stammerers. First of all, to demonstrate the fact that we were 'different', like we needed telling, we first had to take the white tablecloths off the tables in the room and place them over our heads. Like Halloween ghosts, hooded up in white linen we walked around the room repeating aloud, "I am a Stammerer, I do accept who I am". Over half the attendees walked out before lunch time and who could blame them. I'm surprised we weren't thrown out of the hotel for being crazy or, indeed, misusing the table linens! The attempt at demonstrating 'difference' failed. Maybe if they had come up with a better way to explain and practice what they wanted to achieve it may have worked out differently. Funnily enough, years later I discovered that they were on the right track, but couldn't quite put it across.

After the A.G.M much of the confidence they had built up quickly ebbed away. I went back on one further refresher course but it was very poorly attended. However many friendships were made and some of those people have remained close to this day.

My own speech had improved and though far from perfect it never went back to where it was before I went on that course. I felt a vast improvement in my whole self. Just knowing that other people were going through what I went through also really helped.

Over the next few years I tried a few other things but nothing ever worked. I then tried to find something that would involve group therapy, but to no avail.

Eventually when I was thirty five I attended a course that involved group sessions. The moment I walked in the door I knew it was a money-making racket. I had seen the signs before. All the same I stayed and completed the course in the hope that I was wrong; I wasn't. I returned home very deflated and told Monica that there was nothing available for adults who stammer. I would just have to live with it for the rest of my life. I resolved to cope as best I could. It wasn't long before I also had to cope with Soon I would also have to cope with the cruelty of losing someone I loved dearly.

— Chapter Nineteen —

Nanny Evans

Maisie Evans was her name but to me she was always Nanny Evans. My stammering never bothered Nanny Evans and she would stop whatever she was doing and listen to me speak.

"Don't worry" she would say, "You'll grow out of that before you're fourteen, just don't worry about it."

Despite her words I could see it in her face that she was worried about my speech and even though she would attempt to soothe me with her words I would still think of myself as a stammerer and not as a person who had a stammer.

Nanny Evans was a very hard worker, always starting her day before six o'clock in the morning. While her family slept she was up, completing all her household chores before they rose for a hearty breakfast that she prepared every morning. For such a small woman she had bundles of energy.

When I was young she kept pigs, hens and calves and looked after each of them herself. She did all the cleaning out and feeding but because of them nothing was ever wasted in her house. Any left over food went into, what she called, the slops bucket to be used as animal feed. I used to go and help her after school each day. I'd collect the eggs which the hens could lay anywhere but somehow Nanny Evans always knew where they were. She was also very good with pigs and at one stage she had four sows that each had several banabhs, (baby pigs). She rarely lost any. When it was time for the pigs to be sold, a travelling pig buyer would come to the house. He'd take a look and then poke Nanny's pigs with a big walking stick. She hated this and couldn't stand to see her pigs being mistreated.

One day Mr. Barry, a local pig buyer, came to look at the pigs that had been fattened for sale. Mr. Barry was a very tall man and about twenty stone in weight. Nanny was visibly vexed at the way Mr. Barry was examining her pigs. To add insult to injury he then offered her a very low price. It was the last straw and, as she would put it, she read him the riot act. "How dare you offer me such a low price, who the bloody hell do you think you are? I didn't put all that work into these pigs for you to treat me like a fool just because I'm a woman. If you can't do any better then be on your way and stop wasting my time." She said.

Nanny Evans may have been physically small but if she thought she was being taken advantage of she took on another persona. She suddenly became six feet tall and she would hold her own, bargaining with anybody. Mr. Barry immediately back tracked on his original price and after some more haggling a deal was finally done. Nanny Evans was had a generous spirit. When ever she sold any livestock we all benefited. Harry and I always got new toys and clothes and she very rarely spent any of the money on herself.

She always operated an 'open door policy' at her house. With the exception of the winter months, her front door was always wide open. Nanny Evans never asked if you would you like a cup of tea, she just made it and you would drink it. She was also a fantastic cook. I can still taste her brown and current breads and no one has ever made pancakes like her. Her apple and rhubarb tarts were delicious and she always had something fresh and home made to go with a cup of tea. Even though Nanny Evans had a very busy day, she never let it stop her having a chat with the neighbours, the postman, the milkman, the fruit and vegetable man or the bread man. They all stopped at Nanny's house for a cup of tea and a chat and this was how she kept up to date with the local news.

At least three nights a week people came to Nanny's house to play cards with her and Grandad Douglas. We all called him Pops. He was a gentle, easy going man, almost the complete opposite to Nanny Evans. Whatever she decided to do Pops just went along with it and supported her in everything she did. He worked in the Garden Nursery Business all his life and they both shared a love for their garden which was always in flower. To the side of the house they had a small orchard where they grew vegetables and fruit trees. Pops was gifted when it came to gardening.

He also had a great love of music and enjoyed playing cards. Relatives and friends would arrive at the house around 7.30pm on a given evening for a game. There could be as many as twelve people playing at the big kitchen table. Pops had his own black-wooden wrap around chair that nobody else ever sat on. He was joined by Nanny Evans, my mother, Uncle Joe, friends and neighbours. The card games would last until about eleven o'clock with a half hour interval for tea, sandwiches and a chat at around nine pm.

Sometimes a card player would play music. My mother's Uncle Martin, Nanny's brother, was very good at the harmonica and the spoons and if he was there we'd push back the furniture and the adults would dance. I loved watching it and I feel privileged that I was part of it.

The arrival of Television soon did away with that way of life. Nanny Evans was a very progressive woman. She was the first person in our locality to own a television set. People came from far and near just to look at an image of St. Bridget's cross which was the test signal for the new national television station. When the station broadcast for the first time Nanny Evans' house was packed to the rafters with people coming and going to get a glimpse of this miraculous thing called television.

When I was eight years old Pops died suddenly from a heart attack. The locality was devastated because he was well known and much loved. I was eight years old and it was the first time I had ever seen a corpse. I remember feeling quite frightened by it. Pops' wake was held at his home, a traditional Irish ritual. He was laid out by Nanny Evans and a neighbour, in the bed he passed away in. I remember Nanny explaining to Harry and I that Pops was 'only sleeping'. She told us he would sleep like this forever and that he was going to a lovely place. She then lifted us onto the bed to kiss him goodbye.

The wake lasted for two days and one night. It didn't matter what time it was people came to pay their respects, so the kettle was always on the boil. Neighbours brought mountains of sandwiches, cakes, tarts, and brown bread. There was drink for the men, and lemonade and tea for the women and children. Nanny Evans' house wasn't that big so people chatted outside, sitting on walls or steps, standing on the grass at the front, in the orchard; wherever there was space. I never saw as many people in the one place. Pops was laid to rest less then two miles from his home and it was the first funeral I remember attending. It was also the first time I cried without really knowing why I was crying. It's strange how certain things stick in your mind.

Pops' death had, what seemed to me, a strange effect on Nanny Evans. She was working harder then ever in the garden and looking after her animals. Maybe it was her way of dealing with his death but for a long time it seemed as if a light inside her had gone out.

Nanny Evans had very little formal education and she couldn't read or write. My Mother, Aunt Margaret or Uncle Joe would write for her and read any letters or newspapers aloud to her. Yet what she lacked in education she made up for in her wisdom and understanding of life. She was clever and years before her time. She could size a person up within minutes of meeting them and she was seldom wrong.

Very occasionally Nanny Evans would get sick and I would sometimes be kept at home from school to look after her while Uncle Joe and Aunt Margaret were at work. It was during these times that we would talk at length and she would give me valuable advice. "Get a good education, strive to do your best at whatever you do and never sell yourself short", was part of her mantra.

Above all, though, her most important message was, "Enjoy life and enjoy yourself. Pay no attention to what other people think of you. It's what you think of yourself that is important." She said this many times over the years.

Whenever I read or spoke to Nanny Evans I never stammered. I seemed to be in another place entirely, yet if a stranger walked in my stammer reappeared instantly.

Overall Nanny Evans enjoyed good health and didn't drink or smoke. She was the focal point for the whole family, and everything radiated from her. She influenced us all. It was only in the latter years of her life that she had to slow down and take things easy. She loved the company of her Grandchildren and Great Grandchildren and she even had one Great-Great Grandchild while she was alive. She always seemed to have more time for the boys than she had for the girls and she readily admitted this to anyone who asked her, but she never gave a reason or an explanation as to why, it was just the way she was.

Nanny Evans passed away on the 2nd of May 1990 at the age of 79 years. Though she had not been well in the previous few months and we knew she was slipping away from us, it was still a shock when it finally happened.

Society had moved on since Pops' funeral, including the tradition of waking people in their own homes and so Nanny Evans was laid out in a Funeral Parlour. When I heard she had died I took some time out to be on my own. I had a lot of thinking to do. I generally go for a walk on the beach, road, or wood; it doesn't really matter. It is during these walks that I figure things out in my head.

This walk was different. I spoke to Nanny Evans and I told her that I wanted to say prayers at her removal, that I wanted to do a reading at her Funeral Mass, but because of my stammer I couldn't. I wanted her to understand and I knew she would, better than anyone else. I just wanted to talk to her in my own way. I was her eldest Grandson and it grieved me deeply that I couldn't even say a simple prayer at her funeral. It came crashing home to me how imprisoned I was by my stammer.

I was 34 years old and had achieved many things in my life yet, this one thing that meant so much to me, was still out of reach. It suddenly dawned on me that day that I wouldn't be able to speak at my mother or father's funerals either when the time came. That would be even worse than this. Was I to be haunted by this feeling of uselessness all my life? With my Grandmother barely cold, here I was throwing my self into worry about the future, dreading either of my parents passing away.

This is a prime example of how my stammer affected me emotionally. I was tortured by the fact that I couldn't say a simple prayer at Nanny Evans' funeral. I was unable to say goodbye to her the way I wanted to.

Not a day goes by that I don't think of Nanny Evans. Her memory is evoked by smelling fresh baked bread, seeing apple or rhubarb tart, watching a slight woman expressing herself and being assertive and often I'll be inspired to quote one of her many wise old sayings. All of these little things remind me of her. I know she is out there somewhere looking after and guiding me.

The one thing she always wanted was for me to be able to speak well. Unfortunately she never got to hear it, but maybe in her own way she was the one who guided me onto the path that would take me there, the Freedom of Speech path. They say we all have a Guardian Angel who watches over us in our every day lives. I like to think that Nanny Evans is mine.

— CHAPTER TWENTY —

Feeling Useless

I often worried about Monica, Gary or Alan getting sick or having an accident and that I would be the only one there to make that important phone call. My Father suffered from stomach ulcers for a number of years. They flared up every now and then but he had medication to ease the pain. As the years went by they became gradually worse and the medical profession offered no solutions. He was starting to bleed internally and his doctors couldn't find the source or location of it. Dad was in hospital twice for observation but both times he was discharged without ever really finding out what was wrong.

One summer's evening I was cutting the lawn when Monica shouted out to me,

"Come quick your mother is on the phone, there's something wrong with your father".

When I eventually calmed my mother down she asked me to come up to the house as my father wasn't well. My parents lived about two miles away from us so I was there in less than five minutes. What my mother hadn't told me on the phone was that Dad had collapsed on the floor and was vomiting up blood. By the time I got there he was as white as a sheet and so weak he couldn't move. I telephoned Monica immediately to get her to ring the doctor, but when I spoke to Monica she was barely able to understand what I was saying. I stammered so much I had to repeat myself at least three times before she finally understood. Monica and the doctor arrived at the same time and we were told to get Dad to a hospital immediately. There was no time to wait for an ambulance. We carried Dad to the car and the doctor phoned ahead to the hospital.

My poor mother, who was not very well herself was very distressed so my Aunt Margaret and her family looked after her until my sister Marie arrived. The drive to the hospital is nothing but a blur. All I know is that we got there just in time to save his life. Monica spoke for me at the registration desk; I just signed all the relevant forms as Dad needed immediate surgery to stop the internal bleeding. He stayed in the hospital for almost a month. He was a very lucky man and I am happy to say that over time he made a full recovery.

While we were waiting in the hospital I re-lived the telephone conversation with Monica. I felt utterly useless. What would have happened if she had gone out and not answered the phone? How would I have gotten help for Dad? My speech was bad enough on the phone with Monica, what would it have been like with the doctor who was a relative stranger? What would I do if it had been Monica in Dad's situation? All of these thoughts ran around and around in my head, each one becoming a more frightening scenario. What if it were Gary, Alan or Jimmy at work or a car accident? If it depended on me to make that important phone call they would all be in serious trouble. This is another example of how the mere sight or sound of a phone would almost paralyze me. I was like a ticking bomb ready to mentally explode by the common sound of a ringing phone. Even in my own home I avoided answering it. The incident with my father reinforced in me the belief that I would never be able to use a phone. Dad made a full recovery but I will never forget that night when his life depended on a phone call and I couldn't make it. The phone had once again found me out and it just reinforced my feelings of uselessness.

From the time I was a teenager anything that came to my attention regarding stammering always got my full attention. However, when people mentioned to me that there had been an item on a well known television programme about stammering I didn't show much interest. At least twenty acquaintances told me about it, but no one from my own family or close circle of friends. Maybe those close to me hadn't seen it or maybe they didn't want to bring up the subject. Little did they know that I would have been pleased if they had shown some interest in my speech. Then again, I also realised that people close to me didn't focus on it as much as I did.

A few people who I had made friends with on other stammering recovery programmes had also seen the programme and all, except one, were very sceptical of how this new technique for speaking was practised. Some of them said they would prefer to stammer than speak the way the main speaker on the programme did. When I asked about the technique it seemed to be quite unnatural and maybe they were right, that it was worse than stammering.

One friend, though, decided to give it a go. He said it may do some good and he asked if I was interested. I immediately said no. I had become a hardened sceptic about such techniques. I had been stung too often by con merchants and well meaning fools trying to make handy money from people afflicted by stammering. When I was offered a video of the television programme I turned it down. I suppose I knew that if I watched it I'd be tempted to give this technique a try. I just didn't want to face the hopelessness of disappointment and failure again.

There is a natural high when you have been in contact with other people who stammer. Group situations dedicated to practicing a new way of speaking over a few days give you confidence. The environment is positively geared towards you speaking well and, inevitably, you do. This induces a euphoria or natural high and very often false hope. I had been in that state twice before, I knew what it was like. I also knew that the 'high' wore off. I remembered what happened when I came back to the real world and the support of all the other people was gone. Even though I always gave any new technique my best shot, it was a dreadful feeling when you realised that your stammering behaviours, mindset and mentality were never really changed and had come back as bad as ever. I was forty three years old, tired of wasting time and money, but most of all I couldn't face the feeling of being let down again.

About two months later the friend who had expressed interest in doing this new Stammering Recovery Course phoned me one Sunday evening. To say that I was amazed at how he was speaking is the understatement of the century. He had just arrived home from the course and I was the first person he telephoned. His speech was disciplined, not even a hint of a stammer. There was no pushing through on words, no avoiding words; just clear, calm speech. He invited me for a drink the following evening and even though he lived about thirty miles away I said yes immediately. All the next day I couldn't wait until our meeting. I was well aware that he was experiencing the usual post course high but I was still intrigued.

That night I was with him for over three hours. He told me all about the course, the people who were on it, how the course was instructed and that every one connected with the course was a recovering stammerer, including the course instructor. The way he spoke that evening was very impressive. I knew the tricks to look for, but he used none of them. Ordering drinks, polite conversation with other people including strangers were no problem for him. I knew him well enough to know that in the past he would have avoided situations like this like the plague. I was looking at a new man. His speech had certainly improved but his whole being was changing beyond recognition. He had a newfound confidence and I was extremely happy for him.

Despite all the positive signs, driving home that night I was still very sceptical of this new technique. I wondered if it was just the typical seven to fourteen day wonder and then the gradual backslide into the old way of speaking. Over the next nine months I observed him carefully. I kept in touch with him by phone at least once a week and arranged to meet him at least twice a month. I wanted to monitor his speech but I was also getting as much information as I could about the course he was on.

During the first few weeks his speech did backslide a little but it never went back to where it was initially. I was doubly impressed when he refused the free support and backup which was all part of the course. He never went on any further courses and yet he had come a long way with his speech and confidence. The improvements were very evident and appeared to be lasting. He had mostly achieved this on his own. He was given his own personal speech coach to aid his recovery but he only availed of this person's help for two weeks. I often wondered what it would have been like if he had fully availed of the support. He had come a long way without it. Would his speech be even stronger or was the euphoria or high that I had experienced twice before just lasting with him a bit longer? There were many un-answered questions. I needed further proof before I could stick my neck out and even consider going on this course.

He gave me the name and phone number of the man he was given as his speech coach. I wanted to phone him immediately as I had been assured that he was very understanding and supportive. He was a recovering stammerer himself. It still took me two days to pluck up the courage to make that phone call to this Michael Meaney. I shouldn't have waited, Michael was fantastic. He explained how this new speaking technique worked and how he had brought his speech to where it was now by using it on a daily basis. I hung on every word that Michael said over the first ten minutes that we spoke. I couldn't believe how well he was speaking. If he was using a technique to speak, I couldn't hear it. He was speaking very calmly and naturally and what really impressed me about Michael was that he was not giving me a hard sell. He told me straight out that this Technique was not a cure for stammering. He was straight and frank. If I didn't really desire to change the way I spoke then I shouldn't even try the course as it would be a waste of time and money.

This was completely different to what I had heard many times before from other get rich quick merchants who were happy to take my money and never wanted to see or hear from me again. Even though nine years previously I had promised never to do a speaking course again and I had resigned myself to life as a stammerer, after speaking to Michael I discussed it with Monica,.

Monica agreed with Michael. I should only go if it was what I wanted; I should only do it for myself and not because I thought others wanted me to do it.

"You're the important one, do what is right for you", she said.

The wise words of Nanny Evans came to mind,

"Look after yourself. My priority in life was always looking after everyone else".

Over the next two weeks I thought about it and decided to give it a chance. When I had spoken to Michael Meaney I didn't know that I had made contact with the man who would change my speaking life forever. He was to have a profound impact on me as a person and he was a fine speaking role model for me. He would join a distinguished group of people who have made me the person I am today.

It was September 1999 and I contacted Maree Sweeney who was the Regional Director in Ireland for the speech recovery programme called "The McGuire Programme Freedom's Road". Maree was very helpful and understanding. I liked her sincerity and again I didn't sense any hard sell. Having to deal with sales representatives on a daily basis I knew exactly when the punch line for selling comes. There wasn't one. I didn't even have to pay the fee of six hundred pounds until halfway through the second day of the actual course. I was even more impressed. If at that time I thought the course was not for me, then I could leave and pay nothing except my personal hotel bill for the two nights. I really had very little to lose. However I was aware that the programme was the brainchild of an American called David McGuire. I definitely thought that I was going to get a lesson in marketing and selling, because I knew from experience that the one thing Americans like is making money, so despite the positive vibe I was still trying to work out the catch.

At least twenty new people were expected on the next course in October. There would be a Course Instructor aided by about sixty other people who had previously completed the programme and who were returning to work on their own speech and also to help newcomers learn this technique.

Maree explained that I would have to pay for my own hotel bill travelling expenses and food. She came across as a very genuine person. I think I am a very good judge of a person's character and a person's self speak says a lot about them. When Maree told me that she was recovering from stammering herself I found it hard to believe. She spoke in a very calm relaxed manner and, as with Michael Meaney, I couldn't detect anything strange in the way she was speaking. She was also a very good listener. When I stammered or blocked she didn't say a word until she knew I was finished speaking. She didn't even request a deposit. She explained that the Maguire Programme was run by people who were recovering or were already recovered from stammering. Every one I would have contact with would have completed at least one other course. There were no professional speech therapists involved. This impressed me enormously.

Dave McGuire, the founder of the programme, was a severe stammerer all his life and was only slightly older than myself. He had put his speech recovery programme in place and was now helping people all over the world to recover from stammering by empowering them to help themselves by giving them the tools and the knowledge to progress on their road to freedom from stammering. Dave McGuire had set up his programme in many countries. Each region was run by a Regional Director like Maree and all Regional Directors were recovering stammerers themselves.

I signed up for that next course in October which was taking place in Dublin. Maree sent me an application form and an information pack. It appeared to be very professional and I couldn't find any small print, which was a relief in itself. Everything that Maree had told me on the phone was in the information pack. I showed it to my friend to see if he had received the same one. It was exactly the same. I posted off the application form and it was swiftly acknowledged. The wheels were in motion and all I had to do now was to show up. Over the next few weeks I prayed as I have never prayed before that something good would come from this course. At the back of my mind I remained very sceptical about it all.

In October 1999 I boarded a bus to Dublin to take part in what I had decided would definitely be my last Course ever to do with speech. I had worked hard to put the money together for this. I didn't think it was fair on my family to take the cash from our personal savings. In the past I had invested a lot of time and money on other courses, sometimes when we could least afford it, and Monica had never complained or suggested that I was wasting my time or our money. I always learned something from these courses and I met new people who all had their own opinions on stammering. Whether they were right or wrong it was still knowledge. In some cases I knew more about my stammer than the person that I was paying my hard earned money to.

Monica was the only person from my immediate circle that I confided in this time. I couldn't face the looks of disappointment on their faces if it didn't work. I had had enough of those looks to last me a lifetime. On the bus to Dublin I was apprehensive about what lay in store over the next four days. Would all the other people stammer as badly as I did? Would some only have a slight stammer? I had met several like this on previous courses and I wished that I could speak like they did. I often wondered would I have bothered going on any speech recovery course if I only had a slight stammer. There were tonnes of questions circling in my mind.

When I arrived at the hotel the lovely Maree Sweeney met me. I checked in and was told to come to the bar at eight o'clock for introductions and a chat about the course. In a strange way I was looking forward to the meeting. There were twenty five New Students on the course of mixed gender. It looked like I was not the only one who was trying to improve. I found this very reassuring even though bar situations were always something I tried to avoid as I always felt very uncomfortable from a speaking point of view. At eight O'clock precisely I went down. I was immediately engaged in conversation by a man called Sinclair Bigger who told me he was a recovering stammerer and, like me, he worked in the construction business. Alarm bells went off in my head. Why had this man approached me to make polite conversation? Was it planned or was it just a coincidence that he worked in the construction business also? As we chatted I was very aware of how Sinclair was speaking. I couldn't believe that he had a severe stammer before attending the course. Ordering drinks and engaging other people in conversation were no problem for him. I was also very aware that we were in groups of three or four, with an experienced person who had completed the Course leading the conversation in each group. The only people who were having difficulty with their speech were the new people. Over the evening I was introduced to the course instructor, Michael Meaney, the man I had spoken to on the phone a few months previously. I also noticed that none of the people who had completed the course previously were drinking, neither was Michael Meaney. Was this because drink would interfere with their speech or maybe create the wrong impression? Paranoia set in. Were they all being careful and just putting on a good show?

Maree had explained that each of the newcomers would be sharing a room with, what she described as, an experienced graduate. This was a person who had completed at least one full course. At one stage in the bar I counted at least fifty people. I talked to several others who had completed one or more courses. Some of them were struggling a little bit with their speech and I was glad to see this because I knew how hard it was to work on any new speaking technique. A new way of speaking has to be worked on over a period of time.

When I saw that some people were not using the technique as well as others I realised that everyone was at various stages of recovery. Some may have been working harder than others, but everyone that I spoke to told me straight up that they were there to work on their own speech as well as to help the new people learn and practice the technique. What impressed me on the first evening was that everyone was prepared to speak openly about their stammer and their lives as stammerers.

Sinclair Bigger and myself were still in the bar talking, not drinking, long after everyone else had left and gone to bed. Sinclair told me a lot that night. He could tell I was still sceptical about it. On leaving the bar for the night he said,

"Stick it out until Friday lunchtime, if you think it's not for you at least you will have tried it out."

I said I'd give it my best shot. My room mate on that first night was a man called Michael Buckley; a gentleman. I would have the pleasure of his company over the next the next four days.

Michael Buckley had completed his first course the previous March and this was his third course. I was also very impressed with how he spoke. When he knew he was having difficulty speaking he just got back into using the technique and then he was fine. Michael readily admitted that when he was disciplined with the technique his speech was good. He just needed to practice using it more. He admitted that sometimes he got lazy and didn't focus enough. Michael was a very honest and down to earth person. We spoke well into the early hours of the morning about many other things besides speech. I will never forget Michael Buckley for his advice and reassurance about what lay ahead. As time went on Monica and I became very friendly with Michael and it is a friendship that we value to this day.

— CHAPTER TWENTY ONE —

The Course That Changed My Life

DAY ONE

The Course began at nine am sharp. The first thing we were asked to do was answer a few questions which were recorded on video. The video was to provide living proof of where our speech was at the beginning of the course. We would all be sent our own personal copy when the course was over and we were assured that it would not be used publicly for any promotional reasons. The video session lasted for about three minutes for each newcomer. There were twenty five new people and their stammers ranged from severe to very mild. The ages ranged from fifteen to fifty and, if I remember correctly, four were female. Maree Sweeney asked the questions while another Graduate operated the video camera. The questions were mainly about family or hobbies; simple stuff. Some people who had very covert stammers were asked to read out loud to see if they were avoiding words. Maree had the same script to test this. Some people were asked to make phone calls to see how they reacted on the phone. After the fourth person had completed their video I decided to volunteer next. I just wanted to get it over with. In my opinion the first three speakers were very covert; the next person had struggled a lot and at one point became very emotional. Maree was very good in this situation; again she was very understanding and patient. My turn came. I was very apprehensive about some of the questions and I didn't answer truthfully. I only said what I would have little trouble saying. I avoided words a lot and when I look at that video now I realise how much of a cheat and a fraud I was. I wanted the people who were there to assume that my speech was not that bad. I wanted to impress and to hide the way I really spoke every day.

When the videos were over Maree introduced the Course Instructor Michael Meaney. Michael gave a short talk about himself, where he came from regarding his speech and then went on to give an overview of what would happen over the weekend. He told us what he expected of us regarding discipline and why the other Graduates were there to help and support us. He had seen with his own two eyes how this new way of speaking, that we were soon going to learn, had changed lives and he was going to do his best to help each of us change, not only our way of speaking but how we looked at ourselves as speakers as well.

After a short break, the practical part of the course started. Michael gave us instruction until lunch time. The new speaking technique was based on costal breathing. We were taught about the basic cycle of speaking. He explained how he felt and how he reacted to his listener when he spoke, how his listener's reaction would make his stammer worse and how sometimes he would worry for weeks on end about impending speaking situations. By twelve o'clock on the first morning I knew I would be staying for the duration. I could identify with everything. Thirty years previously Sister Monica had asked me how I felt before and when I stammered, it had been the first and only time that I heard anyone talking about stammering from the inside out and not the outside in. All the other courses I had attended always concentrated on getting the physical aspects of stammering corrected such as the blocking, facial contortions and poor eye contact. Here was a man explaining and approaching the problem in a completely different way. Not only was he talking about the physical but he was also talking about the psychological side of stammering. For the first day we drilled and repeated all the new speaking techniques that we were learning. We drilled them over and over again until we got it right. We would break every fifty minutes where we would consume litres of water to stop our vocal cords from drying out. We would say our name, address, and repeat back various instructions that Michael gave to one of the Graduates who sat opposite us in a chair. We were told how important it was to maintain eye contact with this person. A different Graduate would sit in front of us every fifteen minutes so we would be hearing a new voice and getting new advice. They made sure we were all using the technique properly.

The day was flying by. Everyone was making good progress. I noticed that the Graduates who I had met the previous evening in the bar who had been struggling a little were now in full flow with their speech after practicing the technique for just a short period of time. During the meal breaks the new students were paired off with an experienced Graduate. This way we had to keep practicing what we had just learned. It also prevented us slipping back into our old way of speaking. We were given a different Graduate for each meal break. Both of my graduate partners told me of their experiences using the technique and I soaked it up. I could see they were using many of the tools that Michael had taught us. Seeing it hold up in the outside world gave me great confidence.

The Graduates that we were paired off with ordered our food and conducted any other form of communication that we had to do with the outside world. The new students were only allowed to speak to the other graduates on the course as an absolute rule. Michael told us that it had to be this way until we had more practice using the technique. On other courses I had felt my confidence in my speech rise rapidly but it would only take a small thing to knock it. I understood this rule completely. The longer we spoke in the group situation with people who were disciplined with their own speech, the more ingrained the technique would become. This would lead to a stronger confidence and discipline in the new students.

It was already nine o'clock in the evening. It had been a long day and even though I didn't feel that tired, I could see it in the faces of the others. Michael congratulated all of us on how well we had done, and then he said that the new students were going to prove it to everyone in the room by standing up individually and saying their name, address and phone number. One by one, we all stood up to speak using the new techniques learned that day. There was a round of applause for each person from the experienced graduates, who at this stage of the evening numbered close to one hundred. Twenty five people who twelve hours previously would hardly say a word in front of the video camera were now standing up and addressing an audience of more than one hundred. We were all speaking very well. Even though I had been on many other courses I had never seen or heard anything like this, it was really very empowering.

When it was my turn I thought I spoke well but Michael said that I had a small struggle in the articulators with the words Cloone Road and Ferrybank, which were part of my address. He asked me to cancel the struggle and say them again. As the applause broke out I felt very positive. I clearly remember thinking that these were very genuine people. This definitely wasn't a money racket, they really did want us all to improve. Why else would they have been there, away from their families and friends at ten o'clock on a Thursday night? Some had even travelled long distances to be there.

There were further instructions before we went to bed. No television, no phone calls and no alcohol. Michael and Maree were available if we needed to make a phone call so that we would not slip back into our old way of speaking. We had a 7am start the next morning so a good night's rest was in order. During that first day I had listened to every word that Michael Meaney said. I was in absolute awe of the man. The way he spoke and the way he instructed appeared almost effortless. I remember thinking, "If this man can achieve this why cant I?"

Over the next few days I watched him even more closely. This man was my role model and the walking, talking proof that this new speaking technique worked. Whatever he did I was prepared, even at this early stage of the course, to do the same.

I didn't sleep well after that first day but only because I was excited. I just knew that something good was going to come out of this. Like a child on Christmas Eve I couldn't wait until the next morning.

DAY TWO

The new students had an early start and Michael got us back in the groove straight away. He explained the importance of being disciplined with our new way of speaking. We drilled the new method for an hour before breakfast then, just like the previous day, we were paired off with an experienced graduate for breakfast that gave us more advice and practised the new technique with us. After breakfast we went to work on our speech again with Michael giving us even more instruction. Graduates kept arriving throughout the early morning to compliment the graduates that were there from the previous day. Their concentration, patience and rapport with the new students were impressive and genuine. Each graduate appeared to get enormous pleasure from helping us grasp this new technique. With Michael at the helm each stage of the course moved along smoothly.

At noon it was make your mind up time whether you were going to stay for the duration of the course or leave. I had made up my mind the previous day. I couldn't believe what I was hearing and seeing. It was as if someone had flicked a light switch in my head. We were told over and over again that this new technique was not a cure for stammering, but yet I had met people who had done a fantastic job

138

on their own speech by simply practicing this new way of breathing and speaking. I felt that all of the graduates were marvellous, dedicated people who freely gave up their time to improve the quality of life for people who had the same problem as they had. This alone had a huge impact on me.

Only one person decided it was not for them. They were thanked for coming and left with the knowledge that if they ever decided to come back on another course they would be welcome.

After lunch the course moved up a gear. We were allowed more words per breath. When I maintained the discipline I could feel myself improving as each session went by. At times it was hard to maintain concentration. At times I could feel myself welling up with emotion, a feeling I really didn't understand at the time. Occasionally my mind would wander and I would start thinking,

"Is this real or is it a dream?"

The best way I can describe it is that it was like a large weight getting lighter and lighter as the hours went by. It was a truly remarkable feeling and something I will never forget.

In the late afternoon we were paired off with an experienced graduate to do 'street contacts'. Basically it was introducing the real world and testing what we had been practicing. The new students were to observe the experienced graduates practice the techniques out in the real world to show us and reinforce how this new way of speaking would hold up. We left the hotel and emerged into the daylight.

Winston Boyce was my partner and for the next two hours Winston showed me how to approach and engage strangers in conversation. Not one out of the one hundred people that Winston conversed with had a negative reaction to how he spoke. He explained every technique that he was going to use. Winston made it effortless and natural, I watched incredulously. When we returned all the new students had to give a two minute verbal account of how the street contacts went. The confidence in the room had soared and it was great to see how well everyone was speaking. The change in all of us was amazing. Some students were even relaxed and smiling. I had never smiled about speaking before.

We worked until late. Michael had a lot of instruction to get through and the sessions flew by. Before we retired to bed we were given instructions on how to make phone calls using our new technique, which we would put into practice early the following morning. Again our closing included each of us saying our name, address and phone number individually and successfully. I made sure I didn't have any trouble on the words Cloone or Ferrybank this time around.

It had been another long day of hard work but the results were definitely starting to show. I was looking forward to the next day as my head hit the pillow.

DAY THREE

Phone call practice started at six thirty a.m. For twenty minutes before the calls we had to practice our breathing. For a further ten minutes we practiced the speaking technique with our room mates. We then practiced on the phone by calling other experienced graduates who were staying in the hotel. The phone was my biggest fear. I could never understand how a small piece of plastic had such control over me. Of course it was not the phone itself but my belief that the person on the other end would judge me by my stammering. My phone calls went well and I was hugely relieved as this was a real test of this new technique. At seven am we all met for a session with Michael before breakfast. The importance of following the rules and directions of the McGuire Programme were explained. The graduates then drilled, explained and practised them with us again. This session really set us up for the day ahead.

After breakfast we went through more fifty minute sessions with Michael and other experienced graduates. One session was all about letting go and having fun speaking! At another session it was explained to us that stammering was not just a physical problem but a psychological problem also. We were given guidelines and examples of how we would have to change our attitude and thinking regarding our speech in order to fully recover.

This was all new to me, I had never heard any of it before. It was also coming from people who had walked the walk themselves. Eighty per cent of the one hundred plus people in the room were having no trouble speaking. The rest, like myself, were learning this new technique. I could see the merit in what these people were saying when they talked about, intentions, behaviours, emotions, physical state, perceptions and beliefs. You have to take care of the internal feelings as well as the physical external struggle which is what my listener saw. Hearing this had a powerful effect on me. Whatever I had done in the past regarding my speech had only ever concentrated on the physical external struggle.

Today we would prove to ourselves that this new speaking technique would hold up in the outside world. It was our turn to do street contacts with at least one hundred people; complete strangers. After that we would have to give a short speech on a soap box in front of two or three hundred people on a packed Dublin Street, something similar, I suppose, to the world famous Speakers' Corner in Hyde Park in London. It seemed a daunting task but Michael assured us that if we used our technique properly we would be fine.

I was paired with Winston again. Winston and I had got on well the previous day. He was an Architect by profession so we had a lot to talk about since both of us earned our bread and butter from the construction industry. Apprehensively I left the hotel with Winston reassuring me that as long as I used the technique everything would be fine. I approached my first contact,

"Excuse me could you tell me where we could get a bus to the se, se se,-city se,se, se-centre puh, puh, puh -please?"

The gentleman I had stopped told me where the bus stop was and what number bus we needed. The contact had gone reasonably alright but I had turbulence on "city centre please". Winston kindly explained that I had rushed the last three words and suggested that maybe I just wanted to get the speaking situation over with. He was right and the next four contacts went more or les the same as the first one. I was nervous and stressed. I told Winston and he calmly reminded me what Michael Meaney had said about understanding how you are feeling internally in any given speaking situation. Why was I feeling this way? I knew I could do this.

We took five minutes out so that I could focus on my thoughts and internal feelings. No speaking, just mentally clarifying everything that Winston and Michael had said. I started the contacts again. Shop assistants, men, women, groups of men, groups of women; any person I could ask a question to I approached. The contacts were now going well. Winston would remind me about my eye contact, to maybe pause more and, at one stage, he even got me to disclose to at least ten people that I was in Dublin on a speech recovery programme. I had to reveal that I had stammered severely all my life. The feedback was always positive and these strangers couldn't believe that I had a severe stammer. This was very empowering as speaking to strangers was always very difficult for me, particularly women. If they were shop assistants, waitresses, bank clerks, nurses or teachers I would never engage them in conversation unless it was absolutely necessary. I told Winston this and he suggested that in that case I should direct most of my contacts towards women. One lady I met was a former beauty pageant winner. I explained what I was doing and she was really interested. I had a general conversation about the McGuire Programme with her for at least ten minutes. I couldn't believe that she had stopped to talk to us.

The soap box speeches were fast approaching. When we arrived at the location at least one hundred people had gathered around in a big group. Winston gave me advice regarding my speech on the box and what it entailed. He also told me that he was very impressed by my street contacts. I have to admit I was astounded at how I had spoken on the street. Three days previously I certainly couldn't have dreamt about doing it. This was truly incredible.

With five minutes to go to the start of the soap box speeches all the other students and graduates had arrived. The crowd was growing the whole time and it now numbered over three hundred. The experienced graduates were interacting with the general public informing them about what we were doing. Michael Meaney stood on the box and with excellent voice projection, informed everyone what was going to happen. He told them it was not a miracle or a cure for stammering, but a new technique that empowered people who suffered from the affliction of stammering to speak powerfully and eloquently using costal breathing and other techniques which were all part of the McGuire Programme.

The first new student approached the box. He stood up straight, chest out, relaxed himself and spoke powerfully without a problem. It set the bar and so it continued. All twenty three of us individually stood on a box on a main Dublin shopping street on a busy Saturday afternoon and spoke in front of three or four hundred people. Michael was right, it was no miracle, it was down to the practice over the previous two days and the marvellous graduates who sat and worked with us for hours on end. How each new student successfully spoke from on top of that box was the result of this dedicated work. The feeling of support and emotion from the group during the speeches was palpable. Men, women and children cried as several family members of the new students were there to witness their achievements. The emotional bond that exists around a person who stammers is a powerful one and sometimes it is completely overlooked. It is a bond that is hard to explain. It is only when you are close to it that you realise how powerful it is. Our families and friends want to see us improving our speech and it has a profound effect on them when we succeed. It impacted my own family and hundreds of others that I know. Because I always saw my stammer as my own problem and no one else's, I didn't ask Monica, Gary or Alan to come to those first speeches. With hindsight I think I would have broken down emotionally if I had seen them there. Monica was the only one who even knew I was on this course and since that initial speech I am happy to say that she has seen me make many more.

When it was all over Winston and I went for an early dinner. He explained that I was now on my own. For the rest of my life I would do my own talking and never again allow anyone to speak for me. The meal I ordered that day was only the second meal I had ever ordered in my life without having to point at the words on the menu. I told the waitress exactly what I wanted to eat; I even ordered a cappuccino which I could never even say at home, let alone attempt it in a restaurant. It was a very good feeling.

When we returned for the first session of the evening we were asked to report back on our street contacts and how we felt after our speech experience. Everyone was relaxed and speaking well. Michael moved from student to student, the whole time giving positive feedback on the quality of their speech. When we had all spoken, the experienced graduates gave us a standing ovation. Each of them knew how we felt, because they had done the same thing themselves on their first course. There was a positive charge in the room and we were all enjoying it.

At the last session of the evening Maree and an experienced graduate took the new students away to a private area. We were given two photographs, taken earlier while we were speaking from the box in the street. On the back of the photos Maree asked us to write down how we felt before and after the speech. After a few minutes she asked if anyone wanted to read out what they had written although it wasn't compulsory.

A few people did and you could hear a pin drop. Some of it was very personal to the individual but they still wanted to share their words with the group. It became very emotional at times as people spoke about their past and how their speech had affected their lives in such a negative way. A few of them made promises to themselves that they would never go back to speaking out of control again. We all got a lot from it and the bond that had been developing amongst the group was sealed by this session. We knew the journey each of us had taken over the previous days and we all appreciated where we were now. We then watched the videos from the first day and a film of our speech on the soap box; the difference was remarkable. You could see how everyone was changing but not just in the way they spoke. Their whole personality seemed to be undergoing a transformation. I remember standing up in the group and telling them to grasp this opportunity with both hands, especially the younger people. I heard myself say,

"You now have a taste of what it is like to speak in the normal speaker's world. Do whatever it takes to maintain it, use and practice your new techniques".

We all knew that we would improve our speech and you could see that everyone was committed to doing their best. I also recognised that most of the new students were experiencing a high. I had been through this high twice before on previous courses and I was determined to avoid that trap this time. I would keep my feet firmly on the ground. How we spoke in the future was going to be entirely up to ourselves. We rejoined the experienced graduates for the final session of the evening and our instructions. More phone calls were scheduled for six thirty the next morning.

It was ten o'clock at night but the experienced graduates were still disciplined with their speech. I was slowly slipping towards sceptical mode again. I was looking for signs of them relapsing into their old way of speaking now that the course was coming to a close. I couldn't find any. Maree had shown us her own first day video taken three years previously and we couldn't believe the difference. Maree had a very severe stammer and it was at its worst on her video.

Just one more day to go, it had been a rollercoaster and I was looking forward to going home. As I lay in bed that night I was under no illusions. The technique worked but not without a lot of practice. It would be a challenge but I knew with help and support I would do my best.

GOING HOME

At six o'clock in the morning I hit the shower. Twenty minutes breathing practice, ten minutes speaking practice using the new technique with my room mate Michael Buckley and then phone calls to graduates for half an hour made the early morning fly by. The phone calls went very well and I was really pleased.

Our first session started at seven o'clock. Michael got us to focus again on discipline, how to follow directions and more practice. The course was ending at one pm. The morning sessions prepared us for going home and gave us instructions on how to cope in the real world. After breakfast the session covered things like how to push out of our comfort zones. We had to challenge ourselves by deliberately entering speaking situations that we avoided in the past. The importance of attending group support meetings was stressed. We were each given a personal speech coach and the quality of that link could be the difference between success and failure. Experienced graduates gave us examples of how they coped when they left their first course. They recounted mistakes they had made and how important it was not to beat yourself up if you had a bad day. They explained that the support network of the McGuire Programme was there for everyone and it was important to use it.

We were also given lists of phone coaches, not only from our own country, but from all over the world who we could contact twenty four hours a day for advice and support during our recovery. It was all very comprehensive and well thought out. Michael Meaney made one profound statement that really clicked with me he said "nothing changes regarding your speech unless you are willing to make that change".

I knew exactly what he meant. It was my responsibility from now on to improve my speech. I had to make positive efforts to interact in the ordinary or normal speaker's world. No more holding back; I would have to let go and challenge myself if I was to improve my speech.

At one pm the official instruction ended, there was a thirty minute break and then each person gave a going home speech in front of the whole group which included many family members and friends. Stammering can be a very emotive subject and the going home speeches opened the floodgates. It marked a new beginning, a new way of living and a better quality of life for many of us.

— CHAPTER TWENTY TWO —

Challenges and Change

On Monday morning it was back to work and back to reality. I love my job and doing it means an awful lot to me. I immediately told my business partner Jimmy where I had been over the past four days. I also told all of our employees and a few other people who I met in the course of my business during the day. I was amazed at the positive response that I got from everybody; it was like telling a bad secret that you had kept hidden for years and years. Disclosing to people that I was working on my speech was really helpful.

The first day went reasonably well, I was very focused and aware that I had to use my new speaking tools to improve my speech. At dinner that night I explained to Gary and Alan where I had been. They were both very supportive even though I could sense a little discomfort when the subject of stammering was discussed around the dinner table. I explained to Monica and the boys that I had to do certain things to change the way I spoke. I would have to make a lot of phone calls, spend at least one hour every day working on my speech and practising the new techniques that I had learned. They were more than understanding and offered to help me in whatever way they could. Looking back, having that conversation so soon after the course was the most important building block in my recovery. I explained that I was going to give this new technique my best shot, that it would not be easy and that I had set myself a goal of three years. I believed that by then stammering would no longer be an issue in my life.

Because we are a close family I feel that if I had detected even a hint of reservation from Monica, Gary or Alan I would not have progressed to where I am now. I was acutely aware that I was the one who had to change, not them or the world around me. Monica and I had been married for twenty two years and I had known her since I was sixteen. Shortly after we met she became a very important part of my speaking world. The changes I was going to have to implement would impact on her the most. They had far less implications for anyone else. For the first time in my life I would speak for myself. When we were at the cinema or in a restaurant I would be able to order the tickets and the meals. I was aware that I was about to take away her role. Speaking for me had become second nature to her. I was very conscious of this and I was always on the lookout for signs of how it was affecting her.

There was also a good side to the change. For the first time I could order flowers for special occasions and have them delivered, I could book a weekend away and just surprise her; these were the small things that really mattered. Before writing this book we discussed how my recovery had affected her and she readily admitted that at times she found it tough going. Sometimes taking a step back in speaking situations was hard. If you knew her you would clearly see why as she is a great human being with a heart of gold and is a very sociable creature who I can assure you has no problem in speaking for herself.

On the course we had done sessions on assertiveness which, for a stammerer, is the complete opposite to holding back. We were told that sometimes we may have to be selfish in our recovery and that those close to us may resist the changes. This was one of the main reasons I wanted to actively include my family in my recovery. I knew the changes would be gradual so it was important for me to be aware of the impact they may be having on everyone.

My first support meeting in Kilkenny was also in that first week after the course. I was apprehensive and delighted all at the same time. The meeting lasted two hours. As a new member I had to say my name address and telephone number, we then practised all the techniques that we had learned on the course. Twelve of us attended that night and I found the meeting very disciplined without it being over the top. The people who attended were all very supportive and offered good advice. This support group had been in existence for over eighteen months. My course instructor and primary coach, Michael Meaney, was the support group leader. I found my respect for this man increased every time I spoke to him.

The first three weeks after the course I followed all the rules and directions as best I could. We were told to make one hundred verbal contacts a day with the outside world. Most days I was doing two to three hundred between street contacts and phone contacts. Every evening for at least one hour I would take myself away and make phone contacts. I would speak to Michael, Maree or other coaches on the McGuire Programme. This became a ritual for the first three weeks. At the end of three weeks my speech started to slip back. No one on the McGuire Programme could explain why this was happening. I was doing everything by the book, multiplied by two or three most days. If Michael or Maree had asked me to hang upside down from a tree I would have done it.

I never questioned anything I was asked to do because I knew the advice was right and that the people giving it were genuine. It was the end of the third week and I was getting slightly anxious. I phoned a few of the coaches and even Dave McGuire himself but I didn't find any real answers. I started to wonder if the McGuire Programme was really for me. Self doubt reared its head for the first time. All the work, all the practice; I seemed to be going backwards not forwards. It was eight o'clock on a wet miserable Saturday night and I sat alone in the dark watching the heavy rain cascading down the windows of the conservatory. I was concerned because there was no realistic explanation as to why I was running into trouble with my speech despite the effort I was putting in. I was very despondent about the whole thing and I began to think about packing it in. I decided to phone one more McGuire coach, Liam. I explained the situation to Liam about the amount of work and effort I was putting in and how I seemed to be going backwards. Liam listened intently without interrupting me but when he spoke I will never forget what he said. "Michael your problem is you're trying too hard!" He went on to explain that I would eventually burn myself out and that I was not following the directions. The directions were to do one hundred contacts per day. "You are doing two or three hundred, only do what you are told to do", he said.

It has never ceased to amaze me how two simple statements from Liam turned things around for me. The next day and over the following weeks I did what Liam advised. I started making progress again and I haven't looked back since. That simple phone call, which is all part of the support network on the McGuire Programme, was probably the most important. It reinforced in me the importance of having support and backup from whatever course or programme you do to recover from stammering. It was one of the vital cogs that was missing from everything else that I had ever tried.

Christmas was fast approaching. It was the first Christmas where I didn't really mind being in the company of strangers. My speech was far from normal but I knew I was on the right road. I was already looking forward to my next McGuire course which was in February. The coming year would tell a lot about how I would progress. I could start to see a light at the end of the tunnel I had just entered. I still had a long way to go but I knew with the support of my family and the support and dedication of the new friends I had made that I would succeed.

"One of the most important things to recover from stammering is to PERSEVERE".

— CHAPTER 23 —

Feeling Good

The first thing I did on my road to recovery was to part company with my faithful companions the pen and paper. They were with me always. On the rare occasion that I did not have them I felt naked, vulnerable and exposed.

Over the next twelve months for the first time in my life I began to feel good about myself as a verbal communicator. My speech was far from perfect but I was still working on it every day. I attended all my support group meetings which I was glad to see were not pity parties where we all sat around feeling sorry for ourselves. We actively worked on our speaking tools and techniques. We practised phone calls, giving presentations on subjects that had nothing to do with stammering, role plays, job interviews, you name it, we practised as much as we could.

Looking back the support groups I was involved in and the practice and advice I got from them were vital to my progress. In the first year I attended four full McGuire courses. I met new people each time, made new friends, received new advice and discovered new knowledge to apply to my recovery. After the second course Monica started to ask about them. She wanted to know what happened, how many attended, what exactly we did. I explained it to her as best I could and I suggested that she came with me the next time to see for herself. I had noticed that family and friends were more then welcome to attend. At first she was apprehensive about the idea, feeling that maybe other people on the course would find it intrusive. I assured her this was only her perception. The reality was that it was important for people, if they were serious in their recovery from stammering, to interact with normal speakers even in a course setting. Over the next few months she thought it over and agreed to come to the next one. I phoned Maree to make sure this was alright and she was delighted. "The more wives, family, partners or friends the better", was her reply.

Monica was still very uneasy on the day we left home for the course. I tried to put myself in her shoes and I could understand her concerns. She was afraid that the people on the course might think that she was judging them, they may prefer it if she wasn't there. She also felt that it might put pressure on me having her there. What she was to see and hear over the next four days would change her outlook on stammering and people who have a stammering problem for ever. It had such a positive impact on her that she could not wait to attend the next one. Over the following years she would make many new friends, not only those who participated in the McGuire Programme but from outside as well. Monica, along with other normal speakers, has been vital in giving me good solid advice on perceptions and beliefs regarding how they react to people who stammer. I have applied all this advice to my own speech and it is very important that we look outside the box when recovering from stammering. Advice from normal speakers may be just as important as the advice that we get from courses or professional speech therapists. I took this on board. To recover from stammering I had to start behaving like a normal speaker, both mentally and physically. When the course was over Monica and I spoke for the first time since we had met all those years ago, about what it was like every day when you woke up knowing you were going to stammer. At first she was very upset as she never realised that this was how I saw myself and that these thoughts were in my head every single day. Over the coming weeks the more we spoke about it the more she understood how I felt. I was not looking for sympathy but I was glad that another part of the secret living was out of the bag. The first year of recovery had been a good positive experience.

"When you have the knowledge APPLY it"

One of the greatest satisfactions in my life is that I have opportunities to empower others to help themselves. People arriving on courses, and not just the McGuire courses, are sometimes very fearful about the speaking world. It is a joy to watch as these same people evolve over a few days and start to feel much better. They start to accept themselves for who they are and they no longer live in fear of the speaking world.

I had been on the McGuire Programme for about eighteen months when Michael Meaney approached me and asked if I would like to go on a Staff Training weekend to become part of the McGuire support network. I would be evaluated to see if I was suitable to become a Primary Coach which is a personal speech coach to a new graduate of the programme. After that you could progress to being evaluated for suitability to become a Course Instructor, which is instructing a full course of new students with the help of experienced graduates. A team leader would be another way of explaining this important role. After that you could progress to being a Staff trainer which, as the term suggests, is training in and evaluating new Primary Coaches and Course Instructors. The effect of Michael having the confidence and faith in asking me to attend the Staff Training alone was immense. It gave me confidence in my speech and also in my whole self. Over the next few weeks I studied hard and I was really looking forward to the Staff Training weekend.

Dave McGuire came from America to facilitate the Staff Training weekend. It was the first time I had met him in person and he was very open and honest about himself. He was passionate about what he was doing. His goal in life was to empower people to help themselves to recover from stammering through his McGuire Programme which he had set up in many regions of the world. He gave us a brief talk about his own recovery and how he was still working on his own speech, even though it was quite clear to see and hear that he spoke very well.

Twenty four people attended the training weekend. Dave guided us through various sessions during the day and evening. We did presentations and drilling techniques. The whole time we were being evaluated for things like charisma, conciseness, knowledge and technique. He was looking for good role models; good coaches to help and empower others to recover. On Sunday we sat a three hour written examination paper on the content of the book of the McGuire Programme "Beyond Stammering". This was tough going for me as I had not been in an examination setting for a long time. I found the two days Staff Training very beneficial. I came away with even more knowledge. Dave had also given us a lot of information about his own recovery. He reinforced in us that we had to work hard, persevere and follow directions if we were to have any chance of recovering. It would be two weeks before the results were available and the mark needed to pass was seventy per cent.

A fortnight later Maree phoned. I had passed. I was a new Primary Coach and I can honestly say I was really looking forward to this very important role.

Little did I know then that over the next two and a half years I would progress to become a Course Instructor and a Staff Trainer, which gave me even more ability to empower people to help themselves.

"You can't change what you DON'T acknowledge."

When I became a primary coach I put my name on the coach list as 'contactable at any time'. This list is a directory of primary coaches who graduates of the McGuire Programme can contact. The Primary

Coaches are there to advise and to practice recovery techniques with the graduate. Being contactable at any time I knew that every time I answered the phone I had to use my new speaking technique as best I could. This was a very positive move in my recovery and in a short space of time I had the fear of the phone completely mastered. It would be near impossible for a fluent speaker to understand the fearful grip that the sound of a ring tone or the impending phone call has for some people who stammer. In the past if I had to use the phone on a daily basis I can safely say it would have been mental torture. It could sometimes be a very humiliating experience. If I had several blocks during a call I could almost feel the embarrassment of my listener down the phone line. Those days were gone.

It had taken me two years of using the technique before I can honestly say I had mastered my fear of the phone. I practiced using it in as many situations as I possibly could. I never avoided answering it, whatever the situation. I never avoided returning a phone call. It often occurred to me that I was up against myself the whole time. I was the one making as many phone calls as possible by choice. I often wondered if the techniques and all the practice would hold up in a really stressful real life situation. It wasn't long before my questions were answered.

We had started to build Gary, Niamh and Hollie's new home in June 2002 on a site about five miles from our own home. One damp miserable October Saturday morning I was travelling over to Gary's house with one of my staff in the van. It was early in the morning and we were taking the back roads. They were wet from the damp weather. We were in a fully laden van which was also towing a double axle trailer, also full of tools and materials. The road was narrow but I knew it well. It had numerous bends, some of them very sharp. As we drove along I saw a grey car taking a sharp bend about 100metres ahead of us. I new it was coming too fast. The car was still in my line of vision as I could see over the ditch because we were seated high in the van. About twenty metres ahead of us was another very sharp bend and I knew that if the approaching driver did not slow down he would never hold the car on the bend with the wet surface, he would surely lose control. I immediately pulled the van and trailer up on to the ditch on our side as far as I could. It all happened very quickly but for me it was like watching something in slow motion. We were fully stopped when the car came flying around the bend. I could see the panic in the young man's eyes and face through his windscreen. He hit the brakes, lost control of the car and hit us full on at my side of the van. The impact was so great he pushed my heavy van and trailer about five yards back. My first reaction was to see if John, my passenger, was alright. He was shaken up but uninjured, he immediately exited the van and ran up the road to warn approaching traffic. It is strange how people react following a car accident.

The young driver was hurt. The steering wheel had crushed his chest and he also had other injuries. I was surprised he was still alive given the force of the crash. The impact had driven a metal spirit level right through my front windscreen and his front and back windscreen. It had taken off like a missile, narrowly missing all of us. I ran to his aid but I knew he was in trouble. I immediately dialled the emergency number and asked for an ambulance. I gave them directions and told them what I could about the young man's injuries. A doctor came on the line told me what to do. I was to keep the line open and the emergency unit would phone the police. Because it was a rural area the ambulance team kept in contact at all times, as did the nurse who was with the emergency unit. I just did my best to calm the young man down. He was obviously in severe shock as he was shaking uncontrollably. He kept saying, "Dad will kill me" "Dad will kill me", oblivious to his injuries. Obviously it wasn't his car. It took twenty minutes for the ambulance and emergency team to arrive and take charge of things; to me it felt like a lifetime. They had the situation under control in minutes. The police arrived and took the necessary statements and insurance details and arranged to have the car towed away. I arranged to have my van and trailer removed. Over the next few hours I had to ring Monica to explain what had happened and to assure her that we were okay. I also had to phone my insurance company to arrange for a replacement van. I did it all without any problems. When speaking to the emergency services I was focused because I knew that a young man's life may depend on what I said. I had to communicate clearly and concisely. I remembered the nightmares about situations like this regarding my own family. A few hours later when the shock had worn off I realised how well I had spoken to the emergency services which for me was about as stressful as you can get speaking wise.

I also started to have self doubt about how well I spoke; did I speak well because I didn't have time to think? Was I running on adrenalin? I went for a long walk that evening to figure things out. It was no fluke, the techniques had held up under pressure. I was conscious that I was focused and had used my speaking tools. My mind was put to rest. Everything I had done and everything that I had learned had stood up under pressure. Over the next few months the way I spoke during that experience would have a huge impact. The young man spent two weeks in hospital and made a full recovery.

— CHAPTER TWENTY FOUR —

I'm an Instructor. WOW!

Joe O'Donnell took over from Maree Sweeney as the new Regional Director of the McGuire Programme in Ireland. He asked if I would like to be the Course Instructor for the following August in Dublin. He didn't have to ask twice. I jumped at the opportunity and I felt both honoured and humbled that he had such confidence in me. I started the preparations immediately. Everything I have ever done I have done to the best of my ability and this was going to be the very same. I would leave no stone unturned to make sure that the new people arriving for their first course would receive the very best from the team that I would have supporting me in my first opportunity as Instructor or Team Leader.

The preparation included learning from the McGuire manual which was then called 'Freedoms Road'. I had to learn as much as I could so that my team and I could pass this knowledge on to the new people. We would have to share our own experiences and empower them to help themselves. The months flew by and I also attended a course in the U.K so I could get even more experience.

Two months before the course I chose the graduates to do presentations. I included as many as I could. I believed it was very important that new people could hear and see as many people as possible speaking and using the tools and techniques that they would receive to improve their own speech.

Each person was told how important their role was, how they were role models for every new person on the course. I knew by all of their responses that they would not let me or the new students down. They were all conscientious, quality people who you could depend on. They were people who would work as a team with no hidden agendas. The truth was that all of us had walked the path ourselves.

Monica was kept very busy on the word processor. There were many heated exchanges when I would change things on the Course Schedule just as she had completed it, but fair play prevailed and she bit her tongue and persevered. I don't know what I would have done without her help.

The big day arrived. We went to Dublin on the Wednesday evening for the Reception and Course Introduction for the New Students. I was amazed at the number of experienced graduates who had come along. The instruction didn't start until Thursday morning. We had twenty two new people, all just as nervous and apprehensive as I was myself. We started at nine am on Thursday morning and for the next four days the team and I worked with the new students. Joe told me at lunchtime on Friday that all of them had decided to stay. I was so proud, not only for myself but for all the people who had put in such a great effort. The message had obviously been received loud and clear and the new students were more than confident in what they had heard and seen. The course was a great success. I still receive the occasional call from almost all of the new students who completed that course even though at least four years has passed since then.

Your first course as an Instructor is always special. To hear from these people many years later still evokes good feelings in me. It's great to hear that that they are getting on with their lives and that stammering is no longer the issue that it once was. It made me feel very proud also that our youngest son Alan and his girlfriend Barbara came and sat in on some of the course. They were amazed at what they saw and heard. Talking to them afterwards I also realised how proud he was of me and how far I had come with my own speech.

Sometimes we need to hear this from those we love. It makes all the hard work really worth the effort.

Over the next few years Joe would ask me to instruct three further courses. I was as enthusiastic about each of them as I was about my first one. I learned something new from each one and I continue to learn and expand my knowledge about this intriguing subject we call stammering or stuttering. As a Course Instructor Michael Meaney was my role model. If I can achieve a fraction of the impact on someone's life that Michael had on mine I will die a very proud man. I can pay the man no higher compliment and I mean it sincerely when I say that he continues to inspire me.

Joe O'Donnell and I did our first course together. Little did we know back in October 1999 that Joe would become Regional Director of the McGuire Programme in Ireland and bring it to where it is today. Every organisation needs a good leader, someone who is respected and, more importantly, one who respects others. Joe O'Donnell gave me the chance to be a Course Instructor and later to be a Staff Trainer, something I am eternally grateful for. I often wonder where I would be now if my friend in Kilkenny had not gone on the McGuire Programme? Where would thousands of others, worldwide, be today if Dave McGuire, a severe stutterer himself, had not come up with the McGuire Programme? Where would we be if he did not have the vision, commitment and perseverance to keep going with his Programme? Where would we be if he had not kept on going with his vision when the professional Speech Therapy world was pretty much against his methods?

The McGuire Programme gives people, both young and old, hope and as we all know where there is hope people will persevere.

It is very important that I get across just how much the McGuire Programme has done for me. I have met fantastic people and to all of them who I came into contact with in person or on the phone I am eternally grateful.

I know that the McGuire Programme will not work for every one but the most important thing is that you do get help and support for your speech if you want it. If you have that desire, as far as I am concerned, it doesn't matter where you get it from as long as you get it. Check out the various courses, speak to people who have been on them and then decide which one is best for you. My only advice is that whatever course you decide to go on give it your best shot. Please believe me when I say it is worth the effort.

"On YOUR own YOU are alone"

After the car accident and instructing my first course I felt a new inner confidence in speaking. I felt then, as I know now, that I would never go back to my old stammering behaviour again. My speech was not perfect and every now and then my stammer still came to the fore but compared to how it was there had been a dramatic change. The McGuire Programme and what it teaches had done a fantastic job on the physical side of my speech, but stammering or stuttering is not only a physical problem, it is also psychological one. Both have to be addressed in recovery. In earlier — Chapters I explained how I had developed, from a young age, the mindset and mentality of a stammerer. After two to three years on the McGuire Programme I was still watching how I spoke very carefully in most speaking situations. The mindset and mentality of a stammerer was still there internally, I had not let it go. It was at this stage I realised that I had to step outside of the McGuire Programme. It had brought me as far as it could in my recovery and I had to move further on my own.

The first time I spoke to John Harrison I thought the poor man had fallen out of a tree and landed on his head. I was so focused on the physical side of my stuttering that my mind was not open or ready to accept what John had to say about stammering / stuttering. On a course, where I was the Instructor, a presentation was being given on the John Harrison "Stuttering Hexagon". One of the experienced graduates questioned how the "stuttering hexagon" was being explained. A lively debate ensued where the majority of the experienced graduates disagreed with the lady who had questioned the explanation. I was sitting at the back of the room listening intently to the debate. I realised that, although in the minority, this lady had a valid point and that maybe we were explaining John's stuttering system incorrectly.

Three days after the course I rang John Harrison and discussed it with him. I explained how his Stuttering Hexagon was being explained. He listened intently and he said that he would not entirely agree with this method. He believed it may confuse people. I told him that I, in the past had also explained his system in this way because this was how I had been taught to do it. We agreed to put things right. Over the next few weeks John brought me up to speed on his "Stammering/Stuttering Hexagon" over the phone. It was an education in itself. For the first time I realised that I had to work on my own internal emotions, perceptions and beliefs. I had to get to know how I really 'felt' regarding myself and my speech. After six weeks I had to give a presentation to John of his own work over the phone. His response was that if he was at a McGuire Course and he heard it explained this way he would not have a problem with it. A few months later John Harrison came to Ireland to do a Workshop. I found him to be an intriguing man. He had come to terms with his own speech studied himself over thirty years. He was now passing on this knowledge to other people to help them understand their own stuttering system. At John's Workshop I hung on every word he said. I watched how he spoke and how he interacted with his audience. John had guided me to the next stage of my recovery. I was now looking at my whole stammering self as he had shown me the full picture.

A few weeks after John's workshop, Monica and I were about fourth in line in a queue at the local cinema. The line was being held up because someone was having trouble with a credit card. I was concentrating on what tools or what part of my technique I would practice when asking for the tickets. I was distracted by the chatter of other people in the queue. They were talking about getting popcorn, debating regular or diet coke, discussing what type of chocolate they wanted and chatting about getting a taxi home. It struck me that I was the only one in the queue wondering about what 'tools' I would use to ask for a ticket. I suddenly realised that if I was to enter the normal speaker's world then I would have to alter my behaviour further. I would always remain on the outside while I held onto the mindset and mentality of a stammerer. I realised that I was still consciously thinking about my speaking behaviour constantly.

I was so engrossed and focused on what I had just learned in the queue that I couldn't tell you what the movie was about. It was a huge revelation about myself and my behaviour.

Over the next few months I began to visualise myself as a powerful speaker. Visualisation techniques are a common tool whereby you form a clear mental image in your mind's eye of how you want a situation to be even though it may not be that way in reality. I used the technique over and over again slowly changing my subconscious picture. Eventually the subconscious accepted this information and brought it to pass in the real world. You can use visualisation for virtually anything and not just stammering. I now believe I am a powerful speaker, my behaviour in speaking situations reinforces this and the only thing that will alter this mindset is if I go back to my old stammering behaviour. I had entered the world of powerful speakers at last.

I started concentrating on how well people spoke rather than looking at where their problems were. With the graduates I was coaching on the McGuire Programme, I looked for the positives and how well they spoke, before I addressed any turbulence they were having in their speech. I stopped looking for faults first. I found that when I went to McGuire courses, support groups or other courses outside of McGuire in research for this book that I had to take three or four steps backwards with my speech and mentality.

Where I am now with my speech has taught me to accept who I am; to accept how I speak no matter how I speak. I am no longer paranoid or obsessive about it. For the first time in my life I can honestly say that I am completely relaxed within myself regarding my stammer. It is a very good feeling indeed.

John Harrison taught me that the skills of awareness, observation and visualisation, that I had perfected over the years in order to cover my stammer, could help bring me into the world of a powerful speaker.

If you are a person who stammers you have also perfected these same skills because they are all part of a stammerer's behaviour or the stammering system, if you like. By using those skills in a positive way they can help you overcome the problem.

My stammer was both a physical and a psychological problem. When I addressed the two systems it was an incredible life changing experience. To accept yourself for who you are and what you are is indeed a powerful thing. I became my own speech coach first, applied the techniques I had learned on the McGuire Programme, applied the resources I already had and on top of that those that John Harrison made me aware of. I gave myself permission to be less than perfect. When I have a blip in my speech I accept that I am fallible like every other human being after all. As far as I am aware there is no such thing as a perfect human being so why should I be any different?

When I addressed both the physical and the psychological system I finally uncovered my natural speaking self which has enabled me to leave my stammering or stuttering self behind me. I had to experience turbulence in my speech in the real world in order to improve. I learned much by observing myself both internally and externally. I never looked at turbulence as a negative thing. I had to experience it in order to correct how I felt internally and how I behaved externally during speaking turbulence.

It is attitudes, behaviours and feelings which make up the stammering or stuttering system. These are the components which we learn ourselves. When we put them all together they become our stammering or stuttering system and each one is unique to the individual, we have to understand our own system.

In my experience you cannot find an external solution to an internal problem like stammering. My belief is that recovery from stammering will only be found by people who have come to terms with their stammering / stuttering system. For these people who have walked both paths, the physical and psychological path of recovery, stammering will no longer be an issue in their lives. The key to success in anything is action; you have to take action to achieve what you want.

"Remember those who need help and support. Somewhere someone helped me, now I am willing to give it back" Michael O'Shea.

It is the every day speaking situations that matter to me now. Making or answering phone calls, booking a table in a restaurant and booking flights are all small things that are so important. I no longer have to pray morning and night, asking God to help me conceal my speech. Today I thank my God for where I am and pray that I can help and support others in coming to terms with their own stammer.

I no longer avoid people or situations and I no longer waste time or energy running around like a fool when a simple phone call is the solution. I don't have to wait until a shop is nearly empty before I will go in and ask for something and I don't have to leave my own home because I am afraid I will embarrass my wife and family in front of their friends. I no longer live in fear of being asked a question or live in fear of speaking.

On the first of August 2003 Gary and Niamh got married. All those years ago when he was barely twenty minutes old I was already dreading the thought of having to make a speech at his wedding. How things had changed. I was actually looking forward to the big day. It was a beautiful August afternoon. At no point during the day did I allow any negative speaking thoughts enter my head. Monica and I were very proud parents. Seeing your sons happily move on to the next stage of their lives is a wonderful moment, as any parent will know.

The bride and groom looked radiant as did the bridesmaids and the best man and groomsmen scrubbed up well too. The pageboy did his job as did the flower girls, one of which was Hollie, their beautiful daughter and our first grandchild. Many of the people who helped and supported me through my speech recovery were invited to the wedding. I didn't feel any pressure. There were no thoughts that I had to speak well. I wondered how I would have felt and behaved on this occasion had I not completed the McGuire Programme. I know it would have been very different. This was going to be a day when I would put a lot of ghosts to rest; ghosts that had haunted, and sometimes terrified, me all my speaking life. It was a long time since I had looked forward to anything as much as I did to my speech at Gary's wedding. I am happy to report that everything went fine. I applied everything I had learned and suddenly the ghosts departed. I knew I would never go back to the 'dark place'. For the rest of the wedding and the following day, I enjoyed interacting and socialising without any problems. This was something I would have dreaded in the past. As far as I was concerned the whole weekend was over too quickly.

A while after the wedding I was working in a house when a child across the road fell off her bicycle. It was a nasty fall and resulted in a bloody gash over her eye. I heard the child screaming and I immediately ran outside to see what was wrong. At about the same time the little girl's mother and another lady came on the scene. Seeing that her child was bleeding badly the woman became hysterical. The other lady who couldn't stand the sight of blood just froze on the spot. Neither woman was much use to the injured child so it was up to me to make a decision. I had done a first aid course so I was able to console the little girl while stopping the flow of blood. I also cleaned up her face which made her mother calm down a little, but she was still not fully in control of the situation. I knew that the cut over the child's eye would need to be stitched. They asked me if I could bring the child to the local hospital as neither of them could drive. I immediately phoned a local doctor that I knew and asked if she would attend the child if I brought her to her surgery. I didn't want to spend several hours in an A&E Department. Thanks to my doctor friend within an hour the child was back home nursing a black eye and a few stitches. This story illustrates just how my life had turned around. The old stammering me would have been unable to help in that situation. I would have just held back and not even tried.

The car accident, the child falling off her bike and the death of my grandmother are all real life situations that could happen to any of us at any time. It is only during these events that you realise how important it is to have the ability to cope. I am reasonably calm in most situations now that I can express myself. Having the ability to communicate verbally with the world around me enables me to motivate and soothe others. If you are a stammerer it is important to understand that you too can turn your speaking life around. You can be the person you want to be if you have the desire to change your speaking habits.

The experts say that you need three qualities to develop a good habit; Decision, Discipline and Determination. In order to recover from stammering I would add another three to that list; Focus, Concentration and Perseverance. You will need all of these in the early days of your recovery.

"You will never GROW until you take some steps outside of your comfort zone."

— CHAPTER TWENTY FIVE —

Special People

Our first grandchild was born on the 19th of December 1998. She was christened Hollie. I was delighted with this beautiful name and I had no problem saying it because, just like Harry, it started with the letter 'H'. When I first learned that Gary and Niamh were expecting their first child my first prayer was that both mother and child would be alright and the second was, "Please God don't let the child develop a stammer". The same haunting feeling as I had with both of our sons washed over me again. Will it ever leave me? I honestly don't think it never will.

Gary, Niamh and Hollie lived with us for the first four years after she was born. It was a very special time for all of us. It was great having a baby in the house again. Gary and Niamh were proud parents, Alan, my second son was a very proud uncle and Monica and I were even prouder grandparents. Hollie was commanding a lot of attention and getting it. The first year went by very quickly and I couldn't wait until Hollie started to talk. When she did there was no stopping her and there were no signs of a stammer, thank God.

In the meantime Gary and Niamh were building their new home about five miles away from where we live. They were all looking forward to moving into their new house. Hollie was even helping to complete her bedroom and she was very excited about her first night sleeping there. Monica and I wanted to give Gary, Niamh and

Hollie some space and time to get used to their new surroundings so we stayed away for the first few weeks.

About three weeks after they had moved out of our house and into their own home Hollie started to stumble over simple words like Daddy, Mammy and Nanny. She also became very quiet, almost withdrawn, which was very out of character for her. Monica spoke to me about it after she had been over to the house for lunch one day. I had already noticed it when I spoke to Hollie on the phone. It is very hard to explain how I felt. At first I just remember numbness giving way to a huge wave of emotion. I had to be alone to figure things out. Long walks by the seaside and even longer walks on the old faithful golf course of my childhood days helped me figure out what to do.

Gary and Niamh were getting more and more worried as the weeks went on. Hollie's speech was getting progressively worse. I was very concerned as well. Finally Gary approached me about it. I could feel the anxiety in his voice and I assured him that everything would be ok. It was a very emotional time for both of us.

I believed that Hollie's problem was all down to her recent change in environment. She had left our home, where she was always the centre of plenty of adult attention, and had suddenly been thrust into a much quieter life with just her parents. Also while they were living with us Monica was both her Grandmother and her minder and they had become very close. The move also required a new child minder because of the distance. To a four year old these adjustments effectively changed her life; all the constants had been removed. All in all Hollie had suffered a huge emotional charge which had manifested itself through her speech.

We had to take action. Gary, Niamh, Monica and I discussed the best course of action. Monica, Alan and I began to visit more regularly. We would read bedtime stories to Hollie, get her to read out loud herself and recite nursery rhymes. She was encouraged to answer the phone and make regular phone calls to our home and her other grandparents, Frances and Liam. All the while we never, ever drew attention to her speech. Even Hollie's aunt, who was her new childminder, was informed of the process. We insisted that Hollie was never told to 'slow down', 'take your time', 'calm down', or 'think before you speak'. Nothing to do with the way she spoke was to be talked about in front of her.

It was the Summer and usually at this time of year Monica would spend a lot of time in our caravan by the seaside. Hollie would always go with her for a few weeks. Monica was well used to the subject of stammering. Having played a huge part in my own recovery she understood the mechanics of what we were trying to do. After only two weeks at the seaside with Monica, Hollie's speech was back to normal. Her primary dysfluency stage had gone and, thank God, has never returned.

Because we knew what to do as a family unit we were able to take swift action and didn't allow it to develop into a more serious problem. If you notice dysfluency in a child seek the advice of a good speech therapist or speech pathologist, making sure they have experienced working with stammering previously. I have interviewed and come into contact with many speech therapists and few have had practical experience of stammering.

It is very important to tackle dysfluency at its earliest stage in a child.

We were extremely lucky with Hollie, but only because of my own history and what I had learned from the people on the McGuire Programme regarding their own childhoods and their early experiences of therapy. If it had not worked out as successfully as it did and Hollie continued to have problems I would have advised that she see a Speech Therapist.

"The best prescription for recovering from stammering is knowledge. The secret is to apply it"

GOOD BYE MUM.

On the 1st of October 2003 my mother, Aggie, passed away. Her health had deteriorated over a few years and in that time she had numerous strokes and related illnesses. Monica and I were on holidays on the island of Majorca when Gary telephoned to say that that Nanny had been moved from the Nursing Home, where she lived, to the main General Hospital. This was not unusual as Mum would go to the General Hospital on a regular basis for tests and screening. He told us that it was just 'routine checks' and that they would keep us informed of her progress. Over the next twenty four hours the boys rang four times to tell us of Mum's progress, each time assuring us that it was nothing serious and that everything was alright. Monica and I soon realised that everything was not alright. The following day we hired a car to take a tour of the Island. We stopped in a beautiful little harbour to have lunch. After eating Monica went to look around the shops for an hour and I took a walk on my own. We arranged to meet back at the car. The hour passed and as I was walking back to our meeting point I could see Monica sitting on a bench. I instantly knew something was wrong. Another call had come from Ireland. Mum was slipping in and out of consciousness. We both got into the car and headed back to the hotel. Not a word was spoken for at least fifteen minutes and I will never forget that journey or the silence. When we did finally speak, both of us spoke together and about the same thing; we would make immediate arrangements to get the first available flight home. The holiday representative at the hotel was about as useful as a toilet roll in a bath. "No flights to Ireland", was her unhelpful reply. Time was not on our side. Fortunately our own travel agent in Ireland was able to arrange a flight for the following day.

Once we were sorted out I went for a walk on the beach at Santa Ponsa. It is a beautiful horse shoe bay and that evening, bathed in the fading sunlight, it appeared almost magical. I remember looking out and praying to God that we could get home in time to see Mum one last time. For a brief second I could see Mum's smiling face in the setting sun and then it was gone. It was one of those special moments, so few in a lifetime, but one of mixed emotions as I knew in my heart that Mum's time had come and this time she wouldn't recover. The flight back to Ireland and the drive home was the longest of my life. Monica and I hardly spoke, each wrapped up in our own thoughts. We finally arrived at the hospital at 5pm. Early the following morning Mum slipped peacefully away without pain. It almost felt like she knew we were coming and she wouldn't go without saying goodbye.

My father was heartbroken. My sisters Harry and Valerie managed their grief in their own way. I was devastated and I don't like to think how I would have coped if I hadn't spent time with her just before she died. Aggie was a loving caring person and a great mother who always did the best she could for her children.

Over the next few hours I was in contact with doctors, nurses, priests, and undertakers. That evening I went for a long walk. I was on my own just thinking about her and talking to her. I thought about all the marvellous times that we had together. The time we lived on the golf course, the very place I was walking right now. I remembered drawing water from the well, the sheep, the daisies and the freshly cut grass. Thoughts of moving to Ballinamona, Mum bringing Harry and I to school on her bike, picking blackberries to make jam, the train journeys to see Sister Monica, Mum defending me ferociously to the White Coats! All these wonderful memories came flooding back. This was my hour to grieve and I did. I let it all out and right there I was at one with Mum and Nanny Evans again. The pain of her death began to ebb away like the outgoing tide. It was a special time in a special place that I will never forget and I made a promise that night that I was going to keep.

Over the next two days at Mum's funeral I said the prayers at her removal and I did a reading at her burial mass with her coffin less then six feet away. In front of the whole congregation I spoke with clarity and not a trace of my former stammer. Many people there would have known me personally and some admitted afterwards that they were waiting for me to stammer but I didn't.

I couldn't do this when Nanny Evans died and it had broken my heart at the time but I did it for my beloved mother. It meant the world to me to be able to do this simple thing which so many people take for granted. The promise on the golf course, less then forty eight hours earlier had been kept. I loved my mother and she knew it as I had told her many times when she was alive. Even though she's gone I still speak to her every day, as I do Nanny Evans. They were two very special people in my life and although I can't see them, I believe they are still by my side every day.

"Tell your parents you love them, say it and show it often. Someday it will be to LATE"

HARRY

In November 2005 Monica and I went to a McGuire Programme course in Bournemouth in England. A friend of mine, Martin Coombs, was the course instructor.

I had been on the McGuire Programme for six years at this stage and I had been given the opportunity to help, support and empower hundreds of people who had difficulty speaking. In that time many remarkable people came into my life and in their own special way they each left a lasting impression on me.

Over the next four days I worked with a remarkable, courageous and special fourteen year old called Harry. Harry was at the course with his mum, Amanda, who also had a stammer. They agreed to do the course together so they would be able to help and support each other. Amanda was a covert stammerer and Harry could not phonate sounds correctly. He couldn't phonate the H sound in Harry or the Y in yes or the N in the word no. Being asked his name or simple questions that required a yes or no answer were major problems.

Monica and I arrived on Thursday morning at 11am. Martin asked me if I would work with Harry for a while. Harry was very tense and he kept looking towards a woman who sat a few seats away to his right. He'd smile at her and she'd smile back. I didn't make the connection straight away, but it was his mum, Amanda. Harry and I worked together as a team for the next few hours. We worked on breathing and phonation of sounds. We even worked on smiling and exchanged a few jokes.

Harry is an avid Blackburn Rovers Supporter and I am a Liverpool Supporter so I gave him a bit of a ribbing over that. He smiled and laughed and eventually his fear began to evaporate and he visibly relaxed. Now I knew we could make progress. He worked really hard and after we had lunch together we went for a short walk. I talked and Harry listened. Harry was special and I knew he was coming from a place that I had never been.

I had to concentrate and use all my experience of speech recovery to empower this intelligent and courageous young man to speak. During our lunchtime chat we agreed to give it our best shot. Harry had to understand that he was not the only person in the room that had a speech problem; we all had. We were all there to help and support each other. During lunch I met Amanda for the first time. I could feel the love and warmth between the two of them. I also recognised that Amanda didn't want to hinder Harry's progress by letting her feelings show. Harry was still insecure in himself at this early stage and he was constantly on the lookout for his mother. I knew I had to earn his full trust over the coming hours.

By four o'clock Harry could say his first name. By five o'clock his first and second names were coming clearly. Two hours later he said his name, address and phone number. Suddenly his shoulders were lifted, his chest was out and we were catching glimpses of the real Harry. After tea it was back to working on our speech. I had won Harry's trust.

Formulation was hard for him because he had not formulated the spoken word before. We started working on this and he was making consistent progress. Before we finished for the evening Martin asked all the new students to stand up and say their name address and telephone number. The room fell silent. Amanda stood up and I could see the tears in Harry's eyes. A gentle touch, a smile, a wink of the eye was all that was needed to assure him that this feeling was ok. He smiled back; message received, job done.

Harry stood up in turn in front of Martin. Although Martin maintained good eye contact with a smile on his face, Harry was nervous and his body was tense. Martin's experience showed. A few kind words and Harry relaxed. Then he said his name, his address and his phone number without a problem. The room erupted and everyone stood up spontaneously, the applause was deafening. It was a special time for Harry and a special moment for anyone who had the good fortune of being there. Tears of joy and relief were running down Amanda's face and she wasn't the only one crying; even Harry and I were overwhelmed with emotion and the tears flowed freely.

Harry had made the big breakthrough. He had proved to himself that he could speak. It was the first step on his personal speaking journey and he was transformed by it. He was, for the first time in his life, with people who understood how he felt inside regarding speaking. He was with people who could relate to his fear and his insecurity regarding speaking. Just being there was a positive step for Harry. It was good not to feel alone and different.

Over the next three days Harry made great progress. At times he was apprehensive, particularly when it came time for street contacts, but I was his partner and that helped. We got a taxi into the centre of Bournemouth. We worked on his speech in a lovely public park. Harry was doing well. He told me that he liked kebabs so we went and had one each. We really enjoyed ourselves, but I also realised that Harry was becoming dependent on me and this wasn't good for his recovery.

When we returned from our trip I introduced Harry to Colin and explained that Colin was taking him to the next stage. Harry stood on the popular box in the middle of Bournemouth. I remembered my first time on the box. That day he got the best response from the large crowd that attended. A photograph that was taken of Harry while he was making his speech shows a large banner being held behind him by two big, burly McGuire Graduates. In the picture you can clearly see both men wiping a tear from their eyes. This says how special Harry was to all of us who were there that day. Harry had come a long way. Although everyone on the course had done their part and worked very hard with Harry, he himself had the courage to stand on the box and speak, something that he had feared all his young life. He had now conquered it and it was up to himself to keep it going. He would have the help and support to do so. Amanda was

178

so proud of Harry and he was equally proud of her; he told me this over one of his beloved kebabs.

Having worked with hundreds of people who stammer I am often asked the question,

"Who impressed you the most?" or "Who was the most successful?"

I have seen some fantastic life changing experiences in people of all ages. I have seen people get a new quality of life and keep it. I have seen a special young man like Harry take his first steps towards that new life. Of course the name Harry will always hold a special place in my heart and I have known and loved two people with that name. One of them, I have known all my life and I love her dearly, the other fills me with pride and I feel privileged to know him.

"Stammering is behaviour; it is NOT YOUR Identity"

— CHAPTER TWENTY SIX —

Once a Stammerer, Always a Stammerer

Stammering is individual to each person. Some people feel it is the biggest thing in their lives while to other stammerers it is not. Everyone is different. However the idea that "once a stammerer always a stammerer" has been hotly debated for centuries and I am sure it will continue to be in the future. Over the next few pages I want to give an account of why I believe this statement to be true following my own life experience as a stammerer, and my life now as a person who stammers. I have changed from the way I saw myself in the past. I used to see a stammerer first and then a person. It is very important that you do not perceive yourself as I once did. Always remember that stammering is not who you are, it is something that you do! There are different emotions that surround stammering.

FEAR: Fear was the main driving force behind my stammer, it led to massive word and situation avoidance.
Is it the same for you? If so it can be turned around and you too can have a better quality of life.

EMABARRASMENT: I could write several books on embarrassment. Stammering made me look foolish at times, definitely different, and to someone who didn't know me, maybe even insane.

Do you have feelings like this regarding your speech?

TOXIC SHAME: The shame surrounding my stammer was toxic. It was an excruciating feeling. It was like having several deep cuts which could only be felt from the inside. My shame raged, shrouded in darkness and secrecy. I covered it all up but to eradicate it I had to dig deep and find it again, not a pleasant experience. I had to be open and honest with people regarding my speech. I had to come out of hiding and isolation. I had to take action. My toxic shame was so internalised, so buried, that over a long period of time, every single day of my speaking life I constantly reinforced the negative feelings. It is very important to clarify that I was only ashamed of the way I spoke. The rest of my life was as near to perfect as it could be. For me, self acceptance and seeing myself as a person who stammers rather than a stammerer, helped to get rid of my toxic shame.

Does your stammer cause you shame? You have to be very honest with yourself when you answer this question.

SADDNESS: My stammer caused me great sadness.
Did you ever suffer from sadness regarding your speech?

ANGER: I have never felt any anger towards myself or anyone else regarding my speech. I never took part in the blame game as I always believed it was my problem. I would have to deal with it as best I could. I have met many people who are very angry with themselves and the world around them because of their stammering difficulty. I was very frustrated by my speech over the years but I was lucky that it never manifested itself as anger.
Does the way you speak make you angry?

WORRY: In general I would not class myself as a worrier. I take each day and life as it comes but I do worry about my family; my children and my grandchildren. I pray that they won't develop a stammer because I know, better then anyone what a huge emotional drain it can be. It has a massive emotional charge, not just around the stammerer, but the entire family and also impacts on friends and work colleagues.

Stammering / Stuttering is a process. For the lucky ones it will just ebb away, for others it will develop into adulthood with all the life experiences it will bring on the way. Some will be good and some not so good but inevitably it will turn into heavy emotional baggage.

Do you worry about the way you speak?

Do you worry about your future and your relationships?

Do you worry about your children's speech now or in the future?

HELPLESSNESS: My stammer made me feel helpless regarding my

ability to communicate with the world around me. Because stammering isn't the biggest issue in the world and there is little awareness of the difficulties it brings, I believed I would have to live with this helpless feeling for the rest of my life. I have met many people who stammer and who feel unable to cope with life because of the way they speak. I have met people who have attended years of therapy but gave up because the battle was too lonely and too great to carry on. It was only when I took positive action and sought the support of my family, friends, and like minded people that I felt this helpless feeling dissipate.

Do you sometimes feel helpless or feel that you have no control?

Do you feel the road to recovery is too isolated and too great?

There are many negative emotions that surround stammering, the above are just my top six. I'm sure you can think about many others which may apply to your own life. The good news is that all of these negative emotions surrounding you and your speech can be turned around by getting the correct advice, help and support. If I can do it so can you. The only commitment required is that you have a desire to change and you take that first step to action.

For me, the statement "Once a Stammerer always a Stammerer" is a true one. It is not only about the physical side of stammering. This can be corrected as many people, world wide, have proved. However you can never clear up some of the psychological aspects of it. I still look into my children's future or if I overhear someone stammering in a shop I instantly realise that I was in that position once. When I hear a child stammering, it doesn't matter how hard I try to block it out, my subconscious immediately has an association with the way the child speaks. For these reasons and many more I believe this statement holds truth.

For the adult who stammers it is worth remembering that there is no known cure for adult stammering, but there are countless people out there who are willing to share their knowledge, give you support and maintain that support until you have a better control over your speaking life. In turn it will give you a better quality of life. It doesn't have to be a helpless, hopeless situation.

"We are our secrets."

— CHAPTER TWENTY SEVEN —

Yes, Stammering/Stuttering Could Kill You

Before I attempted to write this — Chapter I sought the advice of people who specialise in the field of suicide. At first I didn't want to write about this subject and how it relates to people who stammer or stutter as I didn't feel qualified.

During the research for this book I conducted many radio interviews in Ireland. I wanted feedback from the general public on stammering and how it affected their lives. I wasn't just looking for people who stammered, but also their families, relations, friends, and work colleagues. The people who stammered either wrote or e-mailed me, they didn't phone, but most gave a number for me to ring at a specified time. Family, work colleagues, people who had an interest in stammering all telephoned first and followed up by letters or e-mail.

The feedback was overwhelming. It took a full three weeks to get back to everyone who contacted me and it is still ongoing. I have learned a lot since I first began the research for this book in May 2005. It was an education. I realised that people just wanted someone to talk to, someone who would listen and understand what they were going through. Others wanted information about how they could help and support their loved ones.

For some, however, it was too late. One set of parents believed that if help, support, advice or just someone to talk to, had been available then their two sons and daughter would still be with them today. They were suffering a tremendous loss.

Parents and Grandparents telephoned who were worried about their children and grandchildren. There were countless stories of waiting lists for speech therapy assessments; two to twelve months, followed by waiting lists for therapy; anything from three months to two years depending on where they lived. These were people who could not afford private therapy. There were parents who had been bringing their children to speech therapy for two or three years only to see their child's speech getting progressively worse. No one ever blamed the therapists for this but they were angry with the system. The general feeling was that no child was ever given enough time.

Friends and work colleagues contacted me just inquiring about help and support. They were looking for advice on what to say or do during a difficult speaking situation with a friend or work mate.

In total more than six hundred people got in touch, all responding to radio interviews, all looking for information, knowledge and guidance. I know that if over six hundred actually took the time and trouble to respond there were many more out there with the same issues who didn't. I was only dealing with the tip of the iceberg.

Having spoken to parents I even spoke to some children who were a little nervous at first but they became more relaxed by the end of the conversation. They just wanted to express themselves, to be talked to and not at. They didn't need to be judged, they just wanted to be listened to. They wanted someone to understand their thoughts and feelings. Some of the children sent me poems and letters to include in this book.

Strangely although more than six hundred people responded there wasn't one person from the professional speech community amongst them. Many professionals heard the interviews or at least heard about them, they have told me so, but not one of them took the opportunity to write, email or phone.

I also spoke to many politicians and civil servants in Ireland regarding funding for speech therapy, the establishment of a Centre of Excellence for children and adults who stammer and the importance of having speech therapists who specialise only in stammering or stuttering because it is such a complex problem. At one of these meetings the following statement was made:

"Funding would never be a priority because, let's face it Michael, no one will ever die from stammering / stuttering."

The official must have known by the expression on my face that he had said something wrong. I then told him about the heartbreaking contacts I had received. The first was from a woman who had lost her son. He was twenty four and had a loving family, a good job and a steady relationship. He only stammered occasionally, but it affected him quite badly. He was naturally quiet and very shy and never spoke up for himself. His stammer was one of the contributory factors in his death. He was being bullied and manipulated at work by some of his colleagues and the evidence of this was contained in the letters he left for his parents and loved ones.

I also told him about the lady who had lost her sister who had stammered all her speaking life. She was just thirty four when she died by suicide. Again she had a loving family but her mother had died from cancer seven years previously. Four years after that trauma her long term relationship had broken up. This woman was well educated and had attended university. She had a good job but never the one she wanted. She always felt her speech held her back both socially and in the work place. She felt she would never be loved as a person because of the way she spoke; again this was contained in the letters she left for her family after she died.

There was another communication from a mother who lost her seventeen year old son. He was soon to sit his final exams in Secondary School. He was bright, intelligent and always did well in school.

He was very outgoing, good at sport and mixed well socially. He had stammered since childhood and it was getting progressively worse. His mother and family had noticed that in the few weeks before his death that his speech had become quite turbulent. Again, in the messages he left for his family he said that he could not face the prospect of college and job Interviews. He felt that no one understood how he felt inside regarding how he spoke and that they never would. He believed that his only way out was suicide.

When I had finished I could see that this official was quite disturbed by what I had told him.

"I didn't realise that this could be the case" was his reply.

He was not aware that stammering could be a major contributing factor for a human being taking their own life. Until I heard these stories first hand I was not that aware of it either. Having spoken to professionals and having read a lot about the subject since, I now understand. It can happen to anyone, so it can happen to someone who stammers or stutters especially when you consider shame, low self esteem and many more negative emotions that make up the mindset of a stammerer.

The aim of this book from day one was to make people aware of how stammering / stuttering can affect people's lives. I wanted to give people an understanding. For the few who succeed in taking their lives let us also think about the many who attempt it.

There are countless millions who, at sometime, will allow the thought to enter their minds but few will never act upon it. Stammering / stuttering is a complex problem, the people who are afflicted by it may have other problems and issues in their lives other than stammering or stuttering.

My main message is that stammering can be successfully treated if it is addressed in childhood with the help of a good experienced speech therapist, preferably someone who specialises in the area of stammering / stuttering. If parents, therapists, and teachers get together they can go a long way to addressing childhood dysfluency.

Once the stammering has progressed into adulthood, I believe it can still be addressed. I am living proof of that. It may mean trying out a lot of speech therapies or programmes before the right method appears. It took me many years to find the right people to help and support me. Many of them had been there all the time but I was not willing to let them in. My attitude towards how I spoke and behaved was completely wrong. If you are willing to change and you have the right attitude, there are literally thousands of people out there to help and support you. However, if you are not willing to change and don't have a good attitude towards change no one can help you realise a better quality of life regarding your speaking self.

Get in touch with people who have knowledge of your stuttering / stammering problem; the correct knowledge is the key to a successful solution. Believe you can change your speaking self. It is possible. Believe that you can have a new quality of life regarding your speech.

"Tremendous things happen to a believer".

HELP SECTION

The Day I became Redundant
An open letter

by Monica O'Shea

October '99 was the start of my redundancy only I wasn't aware of it at the time. It did not happen overnight, it was a gradual process, but at the time I found it very hard to come to terms with and it took me quite a while to grasp that I was no longer needed in my husband's speaking life and that, in fact, this was a positive thing.

I have been happily married to Michael for more than 30 years. His stammer never made a difference. It was only a small part of the person I knew and it was never an issue for me.

Early in our relationship I slipped naturally into the role of Michael's speaking voice. This role intensified when we got married and Michael became self-employed. I made all the phone calls; I ordered the timber or whatever other materials were needed for the business. When we went out for a meal or away on holidays I was the one who did all the ordering or the booking. To be honest I never really thought about the fact that I was doing all this. It was done unconsciously and I didn't realise that in the outside world I was talking for both of us.

When our sons, Gary and Alan, came along and started school and became involved in sport I was the one who went to meet the teacher or stand on the sidelines cheering them on because Michael was always busy. He was meeting clients or doing invoices or getting quotes out, or so I thought. I have since discovered that this was not always the truth and many times he did want to go to all of these things with me but he felt his stammer held him back.

He thought he was protecting us, his family, from the shame and embarrassment that he always saw in people's faces whenever he tried to speak. Of course he never told me any of this at the time. If he had we could have told him that his stammer could never have let us down. We loved him and the way he spoke made no difference to us. Michael is a very loving husband and father and he has always put his family before himself.

Over the years he tried many different methods to control his stammer. Some worked for a few weeks but then he would go back to his normal self. In October 1999 he went on the McGuire Programme and, while I say it was the start of my redundancy, it was also one of the best things to happen to Michael and to us as a family.

When he came home from that first course I noticed a change in him immediately. He seemed to be more confident in himself and over the coming weeks I noticed I wasn't being asked to make phone calls for him anymore. He was making the calls himself. Actually we noticed over the next few months that it was getting harder and harder to use the house phone. Gary was eighteen and Alan was fifteen. Being typical teenagers they often needed to use the telephone but they couldn't get near it. Anytime one of them wanted to use it their Dad was tying up the line. We affectionately christened him "the third teenager" even though he was forty four years old.

Both boys understood that it was an important part of Michael's recovery. He had to make and receive calls every night, so they just used their mobile phones. After that I started to notice other things. For instance I would be told that we were going out to dinner or going away for a week-end. This was all new for me and despite the goodwill behind these gestures I started to feel as if my opinion didn't count anymore and, I suppose, out of control. When we went out to dinner Michael was suddenly ordering the food and I would just sit there, nodding in agreement; all the decisions I used to make were now being made for me. Parent teacher meetings, something Michael would have run a mile from in the past were now on his calendar. "I'll go to this one." He'd say. It was the same with hurling and soccer matches. I didn't understand what was going on. When someone has a stammer everyone believes that it only affects the stammerer, but this is untrue.

Michael and I have always made a good team and I believed that I knew him inside out, but I have learned more about him in the past seven years than I did in our previous 22 years of marriage; luckily it has only made us stronger. But back in '99 I wasn't thinking about that when I was losing my purpose.

When I finally got to meet some of the other people who were on the programme with him and understand what the programme was about, things changed. It was only when I got to know them and their partners that I realised I wasn't alone with these feelings. Others had gone through the same feelings of redundancy as I had.

I finally understood that I wasn't being frozen out but it was what each and every person who completes the programme has to do in order to achieve successful recovery. They have to make the phone calls as the phone holds such great fear for all of them. The same applies to doing street contacts and support meetings.

When I saw that the programme was working for Michael I decided to get to know some of the people involved. It was one of the best decisions I ever made and I have met some lovely people over the years and made some brilliant friends.

Do I still mind having been made redundant? Not one bit. I would do it willingly again tomorrow. I am so proud of what Michael has achieved and I know that our sons, Gary and Alan are also in awe of this wonderful man, their Dad.

If you have a partner who stammers get involved in their recovery. It is the only way to combat the demons that make you feel isolated, left out or left behind.

Love

Monica.

A Message for Children

When I was a child between six and twelve years old I stammered almost every time I spoke, however, I rarely stammered when I was with my Mum, Dad or sisters. I never stammered when I was talking to my Grandmother, Nanny Evans, but I sometimes stammered when I spoke to my Granddad. I found this very confusing. I often asked myself why I could speak in certain situations quite well, but at other times I just couldn't get the words out. When I spoke sometimes, it felt like something was controlling me from the inside without my knowledge. When I would try to speak my body would tense and I would get a funny uncomfortable feeling in my stomach. Sometimes I did some very weird things with my face and eyes when I was trying to speak, just trying to force the words out.

I often noticed what other people did when I stammered. I could see their faces going red or sometimes they would look away or even walk away. This would make me feel even worse. People who don't stammer don't understand what it is like for those of us who do. This is why I wrote this book. I want people who don't stammer to understand.

The more someone gets to know you the better they will understand your stammer. When you become more comfortable in their company you may even find it easier to speak. When you do eventually start to speak quite easily around them they may even comment about it. If someone mentions the way you speak it is a good opportunity for you to talk to them about your stammer. Talking about it will make you feel good and the other person will also feel better and gain a greater understanding about stammering.

When I was seven years old my family had a black and white dog called Spot. Whenever I played with Spot I didn't stammer. I could mimic people, famous voices and celebrities and I often did when I was alone with Spot. The words just flowed out of me. When I got angry or frustrated at something my speech did not flow, it was then at its worst. Yet I have met others who say their speech is at its best when they are angry. Stammering affects everyone differently and it is very important to know that.

I found it very difficult to speak in school and easy to talk at home, yet some stammerers speak very well in school but have greater difficulty talking at home or with their friends. I also stammered a lot when I was tired or sick. Sometimes I was very nervous about my speech and other times I didn't think about it. In school, sometimes, I wouldn't make eye contact with the teacher so she wouldn't ask me a question. At other times I thought that the teacher was ignoring me because of the way I spoke. When adults that I didn't know came to my house I was always very quiet, yet if they had children with them I could talk easily to the other kids without a problem. All these feelings are very normal in the life of a person with a stammer.

Did you know that there are millions of children all over the world who stammer? Even if you are the only person in your class or family that stammers, I can tell you that stammering is a common problem in every country and every language.

We are all different and that's a good thing. People speak in different ways. Some people speak very fast and others very slowly. Some people have high pitched voices and others speak in low tones. We are all unique in the way we speak. Just like our fingerprints, no two voices in the world are exactly alike. Just think about it for a second, if we all spoke in the same way, with the same voice the world would be a very boring place. We wouldn't be able to recognise individuals on the telephone or tell the difference between people talking on the radio.

I was always afraid to speak in case I would stammer. In some situations there is no option but to open your mouth and talk. I hope you are not afraid to speak. You can speak properly. You know you can because I am sure you have done it plenty of times when you are alone. I often spoke very well to myself, but when other people were around something happened inside me. If you have these feelings then share them with someone, don't keep them to yourself. It really helps to talk about it.

I also encourage you to look at the things that you are really good at. Everyone is good at some things or many things. Have a look at this list and see how many of these things that you can do well. Running, jumping, football, basketball, drawing, dancing, singing, skipping, computer games, swimming, music, drama, reading; the list could go on forever. Maybe you could add a few more things that you do well to my list right now. You also know that if you are good at something then the more you practice the better you will get. Your speech is just the same. The more you practice speaking the better it will get, no matter how bad your stammer is. If you are attending a speech therapist then make sure you do what they tell you to do. The more you do the better your speech will become. Also the more you talk to your family or friends about your stammering, the easier it will be for you.

Sometimes stammering made me sad. At times like that I didn't want to speak to anyone. You see I thought stammering was wrong or bad. Stammering isn't right or wrong, it is just something that we do. When you speak just let the stammering happen and do not try to hide it. Stammering is just something that you do. If you take this approach you will feel less tense and nervous. The less nervous you are the easier it will be for you to speak; just stay calm. If you find yourself sad or angry about your stammering, that is definitely the time to talk to someone. Talking about things like this always makes the sadness and anger go away.

When I was a child I would do the following when trying to speak:

- Block on words.
- Always block on the first word.
- Close my lips and clench my teeth.
- Close my eyes.
- Tense my body.
- Repeat words over and over again.
- Repeat sounds over and over again.
- Avoid words and sounds.
- Avoid certain situations.
- Never speak in the company of new people.
- Write out lists to hand to people instead of talking.
- Get someone else to talk for me.

If you do any of the things on this list why don't you show it to someone? It would be even better if you made out your own list.

It can be very hard when things keep going wrong and it looks like it is all down to the way you speak. I used to feel like this often and it made me so sad that sometimes I would cry myself to sleep. It is okay to cry and it is nothing to be ashamed of. Crying is just a way of dealing with the frustration and the anger. Stammering can have a very negative effect on us, especially if you are being teased or bullied in school because of it. Teasing can be very hurtful but it is important to realise that children get teased for lots of things in school. Some people suffer because they are considered too short or too tall. Some people get teased about their weight or some people get teased for wearing glasses. It is not right and usually it is the bully who has the problem. A bully will find any number of reasons to pick on someone. This is not right but it happens.

If you are being bullied and teased because of your stammer and it is really hurting you tell your Mum or Dad or someone that can help. They will be able to make it stop.

My Mum and Dad always worried about my stammer. They didn't mind that I stammered but they just wanted what was best for me. I'm sure your family do too. They may even bring you to meet a speech therapist. I have met many speech therapists and they really understand stammering, indeed some of them may be stammerers themselves. They can really help you with your speech. Usually it is your Mum or Dad who will go with you to meet the speech therapist and your teacher may even be invited along for a session. You might get to meet other children with a stammer and you might also get involved in group therapy and other fun activities arranged by the speech therapist. Your parents will also get things to do for you at home and in school and always remember that the more you practice the better it will be. Make sure you follow all the rules and directions that your speech therapist gives you. Think of it like a sports coach or a music teacher; you would follow all their advice in order to improve. If you do the things you are advised to do, you will be amazed at how you will progress.

Do not get into the habit of letting other people speak for you. I allowed this to happen frequently and I often got my friends to say things for me. There were times in school when weeks would go by without a teacher asking me any questions in the classroom. This made me feel very different. Sometimes it is good to ask yourself some questions. Do you like it when friends or family finish your sentences for you? Have you been told any of the following:

- Slow down.
- Take your time.
- Take a deep breath.
- Think about what you are going to say.
- Just stop and start again.
- Don't speak until I say so.

If you recognise these phrases how do you feel? When I was young I noticed that people said these things to me, but not to my sisters or my friends. This made me think that I was very different to everyone else. I then began to think that the way I spoke had to be wrong. This is why I tried not to speak at all. If I was thinking like this and I tried to speak I couldn't get the words out at all. It was only when I was calm and I didn't think about my stammer that the words would come out easily.

If these statements from adults are worrying you just tell them. Talk about it to someone. Your family loves you with or without your stammer. It is not important to them at all. They focus on all the good things about you and so should you.

Think about all the things that you are good at and if, at times, you are feeling hurt because of your speech focus on them even more and speak to the people that care about you most.

It is very important that you always believe in yourself. You are really great just because you are you. Nobody else in the world is exactly the same. This is wonderful. I know that your speech will improve. I have seen hundreds of children all over the world improve their speech and I know that you can do it too. You are a great person.

I am now a grown up and I speak very well. I don't stammer any more. If I can do it, so can you. Best of luck.

A Message for Parents

I am a stammerer, but I am also a parent. I know that you have a natural desire to do what is best for your child. I know that when you hear your child having problems speaking, that it can be a difficult and worrying time. You might ask, "What is the best thing to do?" This book, or any other book, will not answer all your questions, but by reading about the subject of stammering and arming yourself with as much knowledge as possible from books, the Internet, stammerers, and stammering organisations you will begin to understand how complex the problem can be for some children. In some cases however, it is not a problem at all, just a phase they go through. They may grow out of it naturally, but you really can't afford to take that chance with your child's speech.

The question, "Why does my child stammer?" has been left unanswered since the dawn of speech therapy. No one knows for sure what causes it and it appears that there are as many causes as there are stammerers. However one thing that seems to be consistently true is that the initial stammer is actually a result or a symptom of another issue. It is not the root. Following years of study after study the professional speech community has found no solid evidence that it is genetically transmitted, although studies in this area are ongoing.

What they do know is that certain environmental conditions have to be present for stammering to develop in the child and that early intervention is vital in order to prevent the onset of secondary stammering in young children. The research is ongoing and maybe one day they will reach a satisfying answer, but for now that is cold comfort for a worried parent.

As soon as you are aware that your child may have a speech difficulty it is important to see an experienced speech therapist immediately. Do not go into denial or pretend that it is not happening. The sooner you and your child see a professional the sooner your mind will be put to rest. You know your child better than anyone and an experienced speech therapist knows about the mechanics of a child's speech. Together you will have the necessary tools to sort out the problem.

I use the term 'experienced speech therapist' for a reason. It is important that the one you choose has had experience of dealing with stammering in children. Unfortunately it may be difficult to find a therapist who deals exclusively with stammering, but it is very important that you get the right advice and support from the start. If you are not happy with your child's progress after twelve months of speech therapy have no hesitation in finding another therapist. Some parents have had to try two or even three different therapists to hit on the right one. It is common practice to change therapist if it is not working, please don't be afraid to do this.

A speech therapist will assess your child. If they think that the stammer is not a problem it will be a relief. If, in their opinion, there is a possibility of it getting worse then you can begin to address it straight away and they will advise you on the best approach. In the case of children, speech therapy will often involve the parents, family and sometimes school teachers of the child as well. It is very important that parents and teachers follow the instructions of the speech therapist. Your child will not make progress if you don't do your part.

Parents can also help by providing a calm and unhurried environment in the home. Make sure you get to spend focused time as a family every day. Many people find an evening meal together provides that ideal time for conversation and communication without the interference of TV, radio and computers. Maybe you can even make a rule that phones and mobile phones will not be answered during this time.

If your child stammers do your best to wait and let them finish their sentence. Try not to finish sentences or talk for them. Don't rush your child's thoughts or their speech. Slow down your rate of speech when talking to your child or to each other. Try not to look away when your child is speaking. Pause for a second or two before answering your child's questions. A speech therapist will give you much more advice but don't be afraid to ask questions.

Parents may unwittingly do things that can hinder a child's progress. The following is a list that may help you to identify these areas.

- Having a fast, busy environment within the home, giving the child a sense that life is fast and there is never enough time.
- Making the child give little speeches or read aloud for relatives and friends.
- Finishing the child's words or sentences.
- Not stopping to listen when the child speaks.
- Interrupting the child when they are speaking.
- Walking away from the child when they are speaking.
- Requiring the child to speak fast, precisely and maturely at all times. Eg. 'Hurry up' and/or 'spit it out' are very unhelpful phrases.
- Telling the child to 'speak normally' when you find it hard to understand what they are saying. To the child stammering is 'normal'.

The home environment plays a huge role in your child's recovery, just like it can play an important role in their development as a person. It is important to be aware of this. You know your child better than anyone and you will know when they are anxious or stressed. This may manifest itself in their speech. They may be getting teased or bullied in school because of how they speak. This can be very hurtful for both you and the child. If this is the case, talk to the speech therapist and teacher about it.

Your child may want to talk about their stammering. If they do, listen carefully to what they are saying. Some children may not wish to speak about it at all and you might find this frustrating. Again this is a situation where a speech therapist is as much a support for the parent as they are for the child.

And finally,

- Be proactive in your child's recovery and not reactive.
- Seek the help and advice of an experienced speech therapist.
- Get as much knowledge about childhood stammering as you can. Read books or look it up on the Internet. Knowledge is power.
- There are many resources and groups that you can find on the internet; use them.
- Do any practice sessions with your child that are recommended by the speech therapist.

A Message for Primary School Teachers

My main reason for writing this book was to make people aware of what it is like everyday for a person who stammers. If only one person who reads this book helps, encourages or guides a child or an adult with a stammer in the right direction, then it will have been worth it.

Primary school teachers play a vital role in our children's lives. Children trust and respect teachers and some, in their own unique way, even love them. As a teacher you can leave a unique imprint on their lives forever, hopefully a positive one.

Many children have their first experience of dysfulency in the home while for others it may be in school; pre-school or primary school. Stammering is always unique to the individual child and some will only stammer in school or only at home. Please be aware that it can affect children in so many different ways.

If you teach an infant class you know that for some children the transition from home to the school environment can be quite difficult. It can cause a huge emotional charge for both the parents and the child. For a child who has already begun to stammer this change will bring added pressures. They are leaving their comfort zone and although, thankfully, it doesn't affect every child, for some the transition is traumatic.

I want teachers to gain an insight into what may be going on in a child's mind. I speak from my own personal experience and also from extensive research I have done with speech professionals, parents and children aged between five and thirteen.

The first thing to note is that children who stammer are like any other child. Stammering is not an indication of lack of intelligence or talent, they just have a dysfluency in their speech. For some it may be obvious every time they talk. This is Overt Stammering. Some children can hide it very well through avoidance and word substitution and this is known as Covert Stammering.

In some cases a child's dysfluency may not be addressed until the child is in primary school. It is possible that the child never stammered at home or maybe the parents were in denial about the dysfluency in their child's speech. I have come across many parents who were aware of the problem but just didn't know what to do.

If the child is attending speech therapy the teacher should be made aware of this. You may even be asked to phone or meet the speech professional who will advise you on how best to help. It is an established fact that children have the greatest chance of total recovery if the problem is addressed in their primary school years. It has also been noted that success is achieved when parents, teachers and speech professionals work together. Fortunately today there is more information and resources available than there were when I was a child.

For the child who only began to stammer after starting school it is often hard to get professional help. In Ireland there are many reasons for this; lack of speech professionals in some areas, denial by parents that the dysfluency exists, the belief that the child will 'grow out of it', the lack of specialist speech therapists in the area of childhood stammering (even in the private sector) or the lack of communication and long waiting lists within the health service. It may have to be the teacher who brings the child's dysfluency to the parent's attention.

The behaviours of a child who stammers are many and varied. Personally when I was a child I would avoid eye contact and drop my head instantly for fear of a teacher asking me a question. I had notes for the teacher if I was feeling unwell and notes from my parents regarding sickness or days off. I always had my homework done so I never had to explain verbally not having it done. I would often leave a room on the pretext of going to the toilet to avoid speaking in groups. I would get my friends to ask a teacher something. Every single day of my primary school life I lived on the edge, in constant fear of being asked a question in class.

When I was asked a question the feelings manifested themselves physically. I would feel a severe tightness in my chest. I also experienced blocking, which made it almost impossible to take a breath. This often led to dizziness and nausea. The internal feelings of shame and guilt at being unable to answer a simple question were hard to bear. Looking back at my own primary school teachers I appreciate greatly the ones that helped and made an effort to understand. If you have read this book you will know that Mr. Smith was less than understanding. In his case I wrote the answers down in fear of his rejection or another beating. I often think that the rejection I saw in his face and the visible signs of impatience were worse than the beatings he doled out with the measuring stick. Physical hurt goes away quickly, but the mental scars took a long time to heal.

Many stammerers relate similar stories of their schooldays. Some had no problem answering questions in school but others had a major battle. It is important that the teacher gets to know the child who stammers. In time they will open up and talk about stammering if it is approached in the right way. Teachers can also give valuable feedback to parents and speech therapists which can help enormously in the child's recovery.

Some children may use many gestures as a substitute for speaking. Fidgeting, slapping the side of their leg, clicking their fingers and other such excessive gestures can be annoying in a classroom full of children. For the child who stammers they are just part of the vast armoury of tricks they use to avoid talking or to avoid situations where they may be asked to speak. You need to be aware that there is much going on in the mind of a child who stammers. A child will find it very difficult to explain the process in a classroom setting. It is better to speak to the child one on one or with their parents in attendance. Although I appreciate that due to the time constraints of modern life, teachers may find it difficult to arrange such meetings.

It is very important that the child develops positive feelings about themselves as speakers. They must not, under any circumstances, be made to feel different regarding classroom activities. They will be very aware as they progress through primary school that they have a dysfluency in their speech. The stammerer may even claim that it doesn't bother or upset them. It is only when you talk to teenagers who stammer that you realise this is far from the truth.

I have never met a teenager or adult who was unaware of the way they spoke in primary school. Very few had any positive experiences regarding speaking. I am glad to say that nearly all of the primary school children I spoke to in researching this book found that generally their primary school teachers are very helpful in class.

The majority felt that their teachers were kind and caring. Many children told me that they found it hard to explain to adults about their inner feelings around stammering. The following are just some of the statements made to me by child stammerers:

- "How could they understand when they don't stammer."
- "How could I explain the pressure in my head."
- "How could they understand knowing the answer but not being able to say it."
- "Therapists and teachers told me to accept my stammer and accept how I speak. It's easy for them to say, they don't know what it's like."
- "My teacher never looks at me when I stammer, she always looks away."
- "When other kids in my school mock me it is very hurtful."

- "When I dribble and stamp my foot trying to say a word some of my classmates laugh at me."

I could fill five or six pages with these heartbreaking quotes, all similar in tone. For a child who stammers primary school can be a very unfriendly world. They have to adapt to the reactions of new teachers and, in some cases, constant mocking which can lead to bullying and intimidation in the school playground. All the child stammerer wants is to be treated the same as everyone else. For some this will never happen. Fortunately by educating teachers and the general public about stammering, hopefully the life of children who stammer will improve. I'm glad to say that some children are already experiencing a positive primary school education.

Parents and other family members are just as affected by the bullying of the stammerer. One mother told me,

"It is like sticking a knife through my heart when I hear my child being mocked because of their stammer".

Another mother cried for the whole day after hearing her eight year old daughter being mercilessly teased by another child from her class as she dropped her off to school one morning. Unfortunately stories like this are more common than children who encounter positive experiences.

The majority of children who stammer get on very well academically and you will often find that they are very good at sports or anything else they put their minds to. A child who stammers may go out of their way to do well, just to over-compensate for their stammer. I can relate to this as I used to do it all the time just to prove that I was as good as anyone else and that apart from my speech I was 'normal'.

What I have told teachers in this — Chapter only scratches the surface of what goes on in the mind of a child with a stammer. When speaking to teachers I was told that in some cases teachers had less than two hours of advice or education in teacher training college regarding child dysfluency. That is two hours out of a three to four year study course! Every teacher I spoke to had to learn as they were faced with the problem. Some teachers had gone through their entire careers without every knowingly having come across a child stammerer.

If you have a pupil with a stammer you may find the following quite helpful.

- Do not rush the child's speech or thoughts.
- Maintain eye contact at all times.
- Try not to finish the child's sentences or words.
- Try sitting or standing in a relaxed way.
- With a young child drop down to their level to maintain good eye contact.
- Try not to use distracting behaviours such as fiddling with a pen or a ring or look away when the child is speaking.
- When the child speaks well remind him/her of how well they are speaking.
- When a child's speech is turbulent ask the child why they think this is so. Try and get the child to open up and talk about their stammering; how it feels, where it hurts or if it hurts.
- Develop a rapport with the child and let them see that you do not see their dysfluency as an issue.
- Develop a rapport with the Parents and the Speech Therapist if the child is attending one.
- Read any of the excellent books written by Professionals for teachers. Some are listed in the further reading section of this book.
- The Internet has excellent sites regarding stammering and relevant links are printed in the further reading section of this book.
- Attend any of the excellent support groups for people who stammer. You will be made very welcome. Your ques-

tions may be answered here quicker than anywhere else as these people have walked the walk.

- Don't get bogged down in the theory of stammering. Practical application is much better.

Stammering is a dysfluency problem in communication with other people. Person to person or when a child is alone in their own world they will seldom stammer. Just ask them.

A Message for Secondary School Teachers

You don't need me to tell you that the transition from Primary to Secondary school can be very difficult for a young person. What I can tell you is that for a young person who stammers the trauma of transition is even more challenging. Many are leaving a comfort zone where they had friends and teachers that they knew well. They are entering a whole new environment with a completely different set of rules. Along with processing and dealing with all the changes, a young stammerer has the added pressure of how they are going to cope with their speech. They will be concerned with how new teachers and new classmates will react to the way they speak. For any young stammerer the Summer before entry into secondary school will be punctuated with anxiety.

Concerns about not fitting in, being rejected, not being part of the crowd, feeling left out or being mocked or bullied are some of their overriding thoughts. For a minority these fears will be realised and it can be very painful. Anecdotal evidence from teachers suggests that at times stammering can become an issue in class, during breaks and forming relationships but, fortunately, the majority of people who stammer cope quite well in secondary school. In my research I spoke to hundreds of teenagers. The majority agreed that they coped well with their speech in secondary school. We can look at this positively but when I stripped it down I was amazed at how many times the word 'cope' or 'coping' came up. This tells us that at a time when life is difficult enough, the teenage stammerer has an added burden.

At one point I spoke to a group of fifth and sixth year students and also some first year University students. All of them, both overt and covert stammerers, cited a marked deterioration in their speech in the weeks before they started secondary school. They all remembered thinking about their speech a lot more than usual around that time also. Most of them noticed that it was at this stage that their parents brought up their speech dysfluency for the first time. Several had overheard conversations within the family regarding their speech. Some had attended speech therapy for the first time during the summer months before starting secondary school, which they found was of little use as it only highlighted the fact that their speech was a problem and inevitably made them more aware of how different they were to fluent speaking students.

By the time a child reaches a certain age all the physical and psychological behaviours and issues that surround stammering have become ingrained in the subconscious mind. If the stammering has not gone away by the time they reach the teenage years, it will require a lot more than what traditional speech therapy has to offer to overcome the dysfluency. One Summer of speech therapy at the age of 12 or 13 will not address several years of negative subconscious programming.

Along with moving to secondary school there is also the natural and recognised difficulty of changing from a child to a young adult. This period of change is a strange time for everyone, but add to that the difficulties and sensitivities surrounding a stammer and the transition can become almost unbearable. These problems can sometimes manifest into signs of aggression by the young adult, contrary to their personality. This can often be a mechanism to protect themselves from mocking or bullying. That was certainly true in my case. On my second day in secondary school one fellow student attempted to mock me during break time. I instinctively knew there and then that this fellow had to be sorted or I would leave myself wide open to future mocking or bullying. Like all school yard bullies, once he was confronted with aggression, which resulted in personal pain and shame for him in front of his peers, I was never mocked again in school by him or by anyone else. I am not saying I was right or wrong in this approach but it was exactly how I coped with that situation in September 1967 at the age of thirteen. This bully went on to intimidate all those who he saw as weak or vulnerable but he left me alone. Bullies are predators and they see a stammer as a weakness or vulnerability; easy pickings. I was lucky I had the courage to stand up for myself but many teenagers don't have that ability. Bullies haven't changed and they are also found in the workplace.

The modern world has brought new forms of bullying and intimidation via e-mail and mobile phone text messaging, so it is no longer just in the school yard that the problems arise. Jackie, who was just twenty when I spoke to her, recalled secondary school,

"I was mocked in class and at breaks. The most hurtful were by text which could come at anytime. I never told anyone in case it got worse as I knew all the girls who sent them."

Donna, twenty four at the time I spoke to her, remembers getting mocked and laughed at in class in front of a teacher.

"It was in third year and the teacher heard it. She did nothing, I was devastated. I wanted to leave the school but it was exam year and my parents persuaded me to stay. I never trusted that teacher again."

Paul, twenty five, left secondary school at fifteen he said,

"I just couldn't cope knowing full well how every day was going to be regarding speaking. I hated secondary school for this reason alone."

Ryan, nineteen, who had just started college said,

"There were three teachers in my school who took time out to talk to me about my speech. This was always one on one during breaks or at the end of class. I found it very helpful. One day I got two texts saying "The stammering geek has become the teachers' pet." I was seventeen and wasn't having any problems in school. Those texts really knocked me for six, my speech and self esteem took a tumble for weeks afterwards".

Claire was twenty one and had just completed her first year as a speech and language therapy student. She said,

"I am a very covert stammerer. The only people who knew I stammered were my family and speech therapist. I would not let my mother tell the Principal of my new school. For two and a half years I hid my stammer from my teachers and fellow students. One day I was reading a poem out loud when out of nowhere I had a severe block on the word 'Butterfly'. I just went to pieces, I felt I had been exposed, stripped naked, found out. I didn't attend school again until the following Monday. It took me four days to come to terms with being found out. I will never forget the word "Butterfly" I will not say it, even now."

Craig, seventeen, was in his final year in secondary school. He said,

"I was really dreading the oral examinations. I found it really tough doing my Juniors. I didn't sleep for days thinking about them. My teachers or parents didn't have a clue what I was going through. This time it will be different as I have speech buddies in my support group to talk to and help me through it."

Sean who was sixteen explained the following,

"I had a Maths/English teacher who did not like me or, as he put it often enough in class, 'my attitude' or 'your attitude stinks' was another of his favourites, anything to demean me in front of others. To get my own back I used to really go out of my way to stammer as badly as I could. I would even push saliva through my lips just to see the discomfort on his face. I would keep it going until he had to turn away, which he always did. I didn't care, it was a mental battle between me and him. A battle I always won."

Vicki, also sixteen, said,

"My French and Maths teachers disliked me as much as I disliked them. They were the two teachers who constantly asked me questions or to read out loud in class. Both of them knew well that it upset me so much that I sometimes cried because my stammering was so intense. Over a period of time I developed a strategy to get my own back on both of them. To make them uncomfortable and embarrassed I would block purposely on every word. I would push out my tongue as far as I could on purpose, straight at them, as if to say 'Up yours, I'm sticking my tongue out at you, you stupid old cow and you cannot even see it'. In a matter of weeks I was asked less and less questions. I had won my battle with the two old cows. I know, Michael, that you will think I was wrong to do it but it got the result I wanted. It meant something to me to know I could easily manipulate a situation like that without either of the old cows knowing what was going on."

Patrick, twenty and in his second year of Medical College explained,

"In secondary school I figured out an easy way to not being asked questions in class. I would block severely on purpose and sometimes I would pretend to be dizzy because I was not taking in any air. The other thing I would do is just keep silent and stare the teacher down, especially if it was a female teacher; it always worked. I was always pleased with myself that I was smarter than the teachers. Like what sort of dopes who knew I had a stammer went out of their way to ask me questions in class to make little of me in front of everyone else. That was how I looked at it then. Now in college the lecturers are more mature and they don't do stupid things like that."

Again these are only a few examples of the mindset, mentality and behaviour of stammerers, all spoken from the lips of people who either are or have been through this part of their lives.

I could fill another book with quotes from stammerers about this period of their lives. Many more quotes and experiences can be viewed on most of the stammering / stuttering websites.

The student who stammers may, from time to time, show his or her frustration regarding their speech. It can be very frustrating when trying to communicate an answer that you know well but cannot verbally say. The behaviours in class may be very similar to that of primary school; no eye contact, no voluntary participation in class, major holding back (which is a common hallmark of most stammerers), sometimes misinterpreted by family or friends as shyness.

It is only in verbal communication that most stammerers experience difficulty in secondary school. They will have no trouble reaching their potential if they apply themselves correctly to any of the subjects that they are learning. In fact, like me, most stammerers have a tendency to over compensate in other areas to make up for their dysfluency.

When I interviewed secondary school teachers and asked what special advice or training they had received on how to deal with a teenager who has dysfluency in their speech in a classroom setting, none of them could honestly say that they remembered it being covered in any great detail in their training. Some said it would be a remedial teacher who would take care of students who experienced speech dysfluency. No one I spoke to, either a person who stammers or a primary/secondary school teacher ever came across a pupil who had a remedial teacher for their stammer.

The teacher can advise their students who stammer on a number of things which may help the student become more at ease. You will know from your experience as a teacher and good communicator how to approach this as each student is different. However, just by showing your interest and giving advice to help the student you will be of huge emotional benefit. To speak about the stammer in a matter of fact way will also help. The majority of people who stammer, especially teenagers, just want someone to break the ice, to break the conspiracy of silence which sometimes surrounds their stammering.

- In Ireland the McGuire Programme runs self help groups all over the country. In fact no one is any more then forty miles from one.

- Most countries have a national stammering association who will put a student in contact with someone in their area. In Ireland it is the
- The Irish Stammering Association but others can be found easily on the Internet.
- Organisations that help people recover from stammering are growing. The most successful seem to be the ones that are run by people who are recovered or recovering themselves. A list of some of these organisations is in the back of this book although it is not definitive.
- Some organisations have phone coaches who will gladly talk to a student about their stammering.
- Some organisations run open days where a student can talk to other students regarding their stammering.
- Organisations like the British Stammering Association are one of the world leaders in the promotion of stammering awareness.

To bring any, or all, of the above up in conversation with a student will show them that you have looked into the subject of stammering. It will illustrate that you have a genuine interest and that you want to guide them in the right direction. Students, especially teenagers, are very much in tune with the Internet and chat rooms. Chat rooms for teenagers who stammer are available. Young adults from all over the world converge here and share their stories and difficulties. They exchange views and experiences of what has helped or hindered them with their speech. These Internet chat rooms have proved very beneficial. There are also plenty of sites that just give advice and practical ideas from people who have come to terms with their speech and are now excellent communicators.

"It is a proven fact that the way you speak significantly determines the way other people respond to you."

A Message for Speech Professionals

The research for this book started in May 2005. I wanted to write this book to make people aware of stammering. I wanted to let people who stammer know that they are not alone and that there are good people out there who are more than willing to help and empower stammerers with knowledge to enable them to help themselves.

The Speech Professional, in most instances, will be the first person that a child, teenager or adult who stammers has the first contact with for help. You are the people who most parents will have contact with regarding their child's speech.

It is well known and well documented that early intervention for a child who stammers is vital. In this area the traditional Speech Therapist / Speech Pathologist does an excellent job. Stammering can be managed very well in a child with the correct therapy. The role of the Speech Therapist / Speech Pathologist is very important at this early stage. Many parents and children I interviewed gave me ample evidence of this. Parents and children agreed that the child's speech would not have improved without the therapist's help. Unfortunately these parents and children were in a minority. Other parents and children did not have the same view. No doubt it was because their child had moved on to secondary stammering, which, for some, was getting progressively worse instead of better.

I feel it is important for Speech Professionals to read the opinions given to me by those who have been through speech therapy at some stage of their stammering lives.

First let me put you in the picture as to how these opinions and information were gathered. Feedback was sought through the media; radio, TV and newspaper interviews were conducted and I received over seven hundred responses. I also attended stammering courses, workshops, seminars, speech and stammering conferences all over the world and, at each, spent time interviewing and talking to the participants and professionals. I met with many Speech Therapists/Pathologists, Parents, Self Help Groups and Organisations and people who have overcome the difficulty and who are now very good communicators.

The amount of information and data I collected was enormous. For eighteen months I spent an average of three hours per day, seven days a week sifting through my findings in an attempt to distil it down for entry into this book. It was tough going at times but it was the heartfelt responses, particularly from the people who stammered and their parents, which kept me going. Where possible I spoke to people by phone. Sometimes I travelled long distances to speak with someone face to face and sometimes I arranged business conferences and exhibitions around interviewing people. At all times I found everyone to be co operative, honest and warm. It was a very positive experience dealing with people who stammer.

Unfortunately the same cannot be said for the Speech professional Community or the Educators of our future Speech Therapists. Several were quite helpful but there were many professionals who treated me with suspicion and sometimes contempt. I was amazed at how many refused to return my calls or e-mails. One lady Professor who had agreed a meeting on two separate occasions never turned up and didn't bother to cancel the meeting. When a third appointment was sought she just refused outright. This is a poor reflection on the professional community.

First, let's look at some views collected regarding therapy and how it is applied. Most children and parents had great respect for the hard work that the therapists did. They all spoke about how much more could be done if there were more therapists and resources available. They spoke about waiting times for assessments, then further waiting times for therapy. The waiting times varied from three months up to two years. People talked about contacting Private Speech Therapists and that some therapists did not take children who stammered.

Parents spoke about turning up for therapy sessions that had been cancelled without their knowledge and therapy sessions being ineffective because of the time given and the frequency. Some sessions were less than an hour long and only once a week, some once a fortnight. This was blamed on the services rather than the individual therapist.

Children talked about how nice the therapists were and how they found their therapist very easy to speak to after two or three sessions. They were often confused that their speech went back to normal as soon as they left the clinic. Parents were frustrated by this also and I am sure you are all aware of this problem.

Older children, in the ten to fourteen year old bracket, spoke about doing, in some cases, years of therapy and that their speech got progressively worse instead of better. If this situation arose they would lose all faith in what the therapist was saying. One twelve year old girl told me,

"My therapist has been getting me to do the same things since I was eight."

A young boy of thirteen said,

"I started therapy when I was eleven. I have had two therapists in two years, each one getting me to do the same things. Yet I know my stammer is getting progressively worse. I only go now to keep my parents happy."

Ruth and Tom are parents of nine year old Kim, who's had three therapists at the same clinic since she was six.

"When we go to the clinic with Kim we sometimes leave with the impression that the therapists are evaluating us. They constantly look out for how Kim interacts with both of us. Do they think we mistreat her or what?"

This was echoed by many other parents as well.

Clio and her partner Ron said,

"We brought our daughter Rebecca who is six to the clinic for therapy. You could see that the two therapists had more interest in us than they had in Rebecca. They must think we are stupid. We walked out and two days later an inspector arrived at our home from the Social to ask why we had walked out."

Mary who is fifteen said,

"I have had four different speech therapists since I was seven. All of them were very nice and they helped me a lot. I know I still stammer but I know I would be stammering a lot worse if I had not attended therapy."

Phillip who is fourteen said,

"I have had two speech therapists since I was eight. The first therapy session lasted for two years and I did make good progress. We then moved to a new area so I did not attend therapy again until I was twelve. I am learning the same things as I learned when I was ten. I don't find the therapy I do now helpful at all. I know my speech is getting worse."

Parents complained about the lack of private speech therapy and many were willing to pay for two sessions a week for their child, regardless of the cost. Parents of teenagers who attended either private clinics or Health Services' clinics were very aware that their children were not making much progress in therapy.

Ann said,

"My son made good progress from the age of ten to twelve, but in the past two years his speech has become worse."

Tim and Paula said,

"We are paying seventy euro a session for our son Simon, twice a week for the past year. He is now sixteen and he knows himself his speech is getting worse."

All is not well within the Professional Community and many are acutely aware of the lack of resources. Resources, or the lack of, were brought up by all of the Speech Therapists that I spoke to. They are aware of the waiting lists of two years or more in some areas. They are aware of the lack of resources for children, teenagers and adults who have progressed on to secondary stammering. They are acutely aware of the lack of Speech Therapy available to teenagers or adults who leave the education system.

Everyone is more educated today about therapy. They can now access the Internet twenty four seven where they can get information regarding almost anything to do with speech. It is through the Internet that most get advice and get their questions answered. I would urge every speech therapist to get advice from people who have lived a lot of their lives through stammering. These people will gladly give you, and your clients, information about their recovery.

What seems to be missing in the professional world is solid advice from those who have experienced life as a stammerer and are now recovered. I wonder if the Professional Community is willing to go down this path. There are a vast number of people all over the world who came to a point in their lives where they knew that traditional therapy was not the answer for them. They each tried other ways and other means to figure things out. The results speak for themselves, they are now fine communicators. Unfortunately the professional community is ignoring this valuable storehouse of information and experience.

Why is it that many speech professionals did not refer teenagers or adults to other forms of help or support regarding their speech? I am happy to report that things are slowly changing in this area. It seems the younger speech therapists are more open minded and more adaptable to change, when allowed to do so.

In Ireland there are few speech therapists that specialise in stammering / stuttering. I have not met or known one speech therapist that practices as a specialist in stammering / stuttering only. Yet, if you speak to a speech therapist who specialises in stammering you can immediately relate to the vast knowledge they have regarding both the physical side of stammering and the underlying psychological side of it as well. I and many others agree that as a person who stammers gets older the psychological issues need to be particularly addressed.

Some speech therapists will not take clients who stammer. Is it because stammering is too time consuming? Is it because the new generation of speech therapists realise that they do not have the right tools, approach or resources to deal with stammering? Maybe it is better to moan about the lack of resources and let people stammer. Let the person who stammers find their own way out of it.

The role of the speech and language therapist is forever evolving. We now live in a modern world where research and communication is very fast. The research into why people stammer is constant, but there is much less emphasis on research into what will help people who experience dysfluency. In some countries therapists are dealing with stammering the way they were taught in college or university many, many, years ago. Things have moved on. Research into why people stammer is of little use to the child, teenager or adult who lives with a stammer day in and day out. Hopefully in time the researchers will find the reason why people stammer and they will come up with a cure or something to prevent it. For now therapists and people like me in the area of self help have to deal with what is presently available. We need to empower people to use the methods that we definitely know will help people to recover from stammering.

The area of self help organisations and support groups for people who stammer are on the increase world wide. Many of these organisations were started by people who believe that stammering and how it is approached is a specialised field. It has to be addressed in a certain way using good back up and support over a period of time. Most important of all is to give the person who stammers a better understanding of the components that cause them to stammer. They must be given the knowledge and tools to apply to their speech. They need encouragement and support on their path to a new speaking life which will inevitably give them a new quality of life.

Speech therapists informed me that they would love to establish a network of support groups for their clients. This is a proven idea and, as we all know has worked for many other situations outside of stammering. In a support group you share experiences, knowledge and in some cases, people who have benefited greatly still attend to support others. People who are taking the self help route are finding it a very good way to deal with their stammering. In the organisation that I am involved with we hold courses every three months. I see people attending over a period of time reach a stage where communication with the world around them is no longer an issue. They, for the most part, have left their stammering issues behind them.

Many years ago the medical profession realised that people with a drink problem needed a support network. Somewhere people could go and get the support and advice that they needed to recover from alcohol addiction. Groups like Alcoholics Anonymous were established to bring people together to help and empower each other to recover. The system has been used for gambling, drug addiction, depression, victims of crime, cancer patients; the list is endless. I believe that in the future a lot more self help organisations and therapists, who specialise in stammering / stuttering only, will come on stream. The traditional speech therapy approach has largely failed most people who are now adult stammerers. Either the approach was wrong or many people fell through the net as children, leaving it too late for the traditional approach to work effectively.

Academics and scientists often set about proving things about stammering. It is impressive research and may lead to greater respect from their peers or secure another round of funding for more research. Unfortunately in the past fifty years very few of these activities have resulted in help or new information for therapists or stammerers. The other difficulty with highbrow research is that the ordinary person who stammers has little understanding of it, no matter how well it has been received at an academic conference. More funding is needed for proven areas of help and support for children and adults who stammer.

Based on my own life's experiences I have come to the conclusion that it is crazy for the professional community to virtually ignore people that have lived through, and recovered from, stammering. I believe that if you need to do or achieve something it is much easier if you speak to people who have done the same thing before you and find out how they did it.

When I look back on my stammering life I realise that I was doing the same things every day regarding my speech and expecting a different result, it couldn't possibly have work. It was not until I met people who gave me new knowledge and guided me in a different direction that things began to change.

If you are a speech professional and you are doing the same therapy with your clients over and over and they do are not responding, surely it is time to look for a different approach or refer the client to something else. If a doctor doesn't know what is wrong with a patient he /she will refer the patient to a specialist for assessment and treatment.

The defining thing for me with any speech professional is seeing a passion in them for their work? This enthusiasm will always shine through. To certain speech professionals it is not just a job and they never allow resources to hold them back, they move on with their clients. These same therapists get results because of this zeal and they are great people, unfortunately it is the clients who suffer when they meet a poor speech professional.

This is my truth based on my world and my experiences of stammering for over forty years. I acknowledge the fact, however, that it is difficult for most speech professionals as they have never had to live the everyday life of a person who stammers/stutters!

Definition of Crazy: Doing the same thing every day and expecting a different result.

REVIEWS

Michael,

Well I told you I would try and finish your book this weekend, but the truth is I couldn't wait! I had the day off today and it was raining outside which made a perfect time to sit out on my balcony, settle in and read. I couldn't put it down. It's absolutely uncanny the way that our lives were unfolding in parallel. We are close to the same age although I am a bit older. While many of us have "The same story" as regards our stuttering, your experiences and feelings were as close to mine from the teen years (I did not attend catholic or church schools) as anyone I have ever heard. I literally had tears running down my face as I relived through your words much of my own pain.

In addition, your sense of independence, individualism and de-termination also mimicked mine. I think, like you, I was athletic, had many friends and led a pretty normal life with the gripping fear and avoidances that lived inside of me every step of the way. The de-scription of you and Monica's early struggles with starting a career were especially poignant. I laughed and reminisced with youJ. Those were difficult and often scary years but we made it!

I pursued my dream of becoming a Veterinarian in spite of my stutter and in spite of the many obstacles; often self imposed. None of the traditional or desperate treatments, I even tried Scientology for a while because they said they could cure me, were very success-ful. Ultimately I found my way out of the forest with the right kind of help at the right time. Your story is an important one to tell. It reinforces my belief that there are many paths out of the forest. It is important that we continue to encourage our comrades affected by stuttering to never give up. Some will discover the path that you followed, others mine and still others a path that neither of us are familiar with yet. The good news is that in finding our voices we created opportunities to travel, to speak and to meet some of the most wonderful people in the world!

A quick note to Monica, thank you for your contribution on "Redundancy". I think your message is invaluable to spouses and other friends and family members of the rest of us who have "found their voice". As you observed, and shared so beautifully, we do go through a significant period of change when we are finally able to say what we want to say when we want to and how we want to. The skills that others learn about turn taking and the art of polite conversation were never necessary for us, for obvious reasons. It takes a while to learn these skills and it can be uncomfortable and bewildering to our loved ones and friends. During the early stages of my recovery one friend said to me when I was being a little too talkative. "You know R****S, I liked you a lot more when you stuttered!" At any rate I think your message will be very enlightening and helpful to many.

Thanks for writing this book, Michael. It is a contribution to the cause, helping those who stutter, their families and professionals.

Be well,

L.R. (U.S.A)

CONTRIBUTIONS

From child to teenage.

He was born in 1938 just before the start of World War II. From the age of four he knew there was something different about himself. When excitement came he got tongue tied. His face would twist and words would not come out. His parents tried to find a cure, but this was 1942 and there were no facilities in place then for children with speaking difficulties. When he was eight years old his father died, so that made a big change in the house; money was really scarce and life was a lot tougher. At school teachers were kind and did not ask him to speak for which he was grateful. Then he began to wonder if they thought that he was retarded or didn't have a brain, but because he was unable to ask, he just let things drift on as they were and stayed quiet and out of the way. Books were a life line where he could find peace and he became an avid reader. At sport he did not take part, especially team games because to call for a pass he could not. So he lived out his school life in solitude and self imposed isolation.

Teenage to marriage.

At fourteen a job was found for him in a shoe factory which he liked because talking was not allowed and he was happy with that. So for eighteen years he worked there. These were the **if only** years when he began to realize what the stammer really meant and he would say (to himself) if only I could speak I could do this or do that. I could chat up girls, join the army or the guards (Gardai), get a better education; there were so many things that could be done and so many doors would open, if only. Then he met a girl and, mostly through notes and the help of a very good friend, they fell in love. He found that he could speak with her and that she respected him and his impediment. Life took on a new meaning and he became more open with people and started to go out more so life was good and the world was a beautiful place. For three years they went out together with long walks and talks and then much to his amazement she said she would marry him. Now came a big obstacle! How would he speak at the marriage ceremony and the wedding breakfast? He knew that there was no way that he could stand up and talk, so the best man filled in for him and the day dragged out and then it was over. He knew himself to be so lucky as to be married as he thought he never would.

Marriage to Retirement.

Life took on a new meaning now, there was someone there all the time who understood and who would wait to hear what he had to say and could really communicate with him. They made plans and dreams together and life was bliss. Then life got better, if it could, as a family came along and now he had his own children to talk to. There was no bother talking to them because they never questioned why he stammered. They just took it as it came and so with the years it became easier to mix and speak. He found that he did not really care so much any more what people thought and that in itself there was an easing of the tension that was causing the stammer in the first place. But still, there was always a wish to be like other people and stand up and speak his mind if he wanted to. Then one night he saw a programme on TV about stammering and decided that at sixty years of age to have one last go at getting rid of this curse that had hung over him all his life and caused him so much pain and misery. So off he went to the course and found, much to his amazement, that there were a lot of other people with a stammer. There he learned that to speak, he would have to keep in mind that he was a stammerer and for fluent speaking to slow down his mind, because it wanted him to say words his mouth was not yet ready for and so he learned to control his breathing by taking full ......breaths and also to control his emotions and the impulse to rush in and speak before he was ready, now it was pause breath, and speak.

Retirement.

Now nearing seventy he finds that he is not a bit bothered by what people think or how they behave towards him. If they want to engage with him, that's great. If not, no big deal. Also how lucky is he that he just has a stammer, which if he applies himself and follows the advice of the people on the course, he can control it. When he looks around and sees the things other people have to suffer he can thank God for what he has. He can see the trees and flowers, hear the birds sing, get up and walk where he likes and so much more. What's a little stammer!

P.M.

A Stutter

Some call it a stammer to make it sound nice.
Some call it a stutter which is more to the point
But whatever it's called, it's really a curse.
It rules your life and makes it worse.
The build up of fear that seizes your brain
when someone turns and asks you your name.
To run, to escape, to leave this behind
but you know that you can't and its got to be said,
sometimes you think, God I wish I was dead.

You want to say something.
And you know words won't come.
So you just stand there and act like you are dumb.
In youth you tasted the pain and frustration.
Of loneliness and isolation.
Oh what you would give to have a voice,
to butt in and have a choice.
To speak and dominate a conversation
instead of listening with building frustration.

But you are careful with your words.
They could turn like sharpened swords.
To pierce the confidence you had found
and grind it cruelly into the ground.
So you may go and seek again
to find strength to overcome the pain
of cruel and unfeeling folk
who look on your impediment as a joke.
But you have got to smile and look away
because you will get this kick most every day.

Some days you're fine and you get by
without a stoppage to mar your sky.
But when you think the next will be as good
something happens to change your mood.
The brain takes off and you lose control
the breathings gone right down the hole.
So you're back, right in the gutter.
With this stupid, stupid stutter!

P.M.

Loss of Innocence

I was seven, I believe, when I became aware that I was a "Stutterer".

Although I have met people who are able to remember the name of every teacher and every classmate they have had since they started school, I have never been able to do so. I think the name of my Grade two teacher was "Miss Woods ", but I do remember well that she brought a tape recorder to school one morning, a morning that was to change my life.

The second grade classroom in St Vincent's Boys School, so many years ago was of medium size and contained about thirty desks arranged in five rows. The students were seated in alphabetical order starting with the "A"s next to the door, at the right front of the room. With a last name starting with "H", I was seated about halfway up the third aisle. The hanging incandescent lights were only bright enough to illuminate the long blackboards mounted on the front and right hand side walls. Additional light came from the row of windows along the left wall.

Entering the classroom that sunny morning, we saw a device on Miss Woods' desk. It was a large reel to reel tape recorder, gray in color with a snap down lid cover, now removed to reveal the disks, dials, wires and a fairly large microphone. Standing next to the teacher's desk was a tall microphone stand which shone bright and silvery from the reflected light. Of course we kids all gathered round this new contraption and wondered what it was there for. Miss Woods told us that she had a "treat" for us and that we would find out what it was later in the morning. We were all disappointed at the delay because we wanted to start playing with this new toy right away.

Finally, after that morning's routine work was completed, our teacher asked us to put the rest of our books away and to get out our readers. Starting with the first seat in the first row, we were to come up to the microphone at the head of the classroom. Each of us was to recite our name and read a passage of poetry out of our texts, about four lines per student. I remember a feeling of anticipation rather then apprehension as I awaited my turn at the tape recorder. Like most of the other students I had never used one before and I was looking forward to this new adventure.

One by one my classmates carried their readers up to the front of the class and stood before the silver microphone stand. Miss Woods had just adjusted the stand so that it was low enough to suit most of the kids and only a slight push was needed to point the microphone in the right direction to accommodate the small difference in size of seven and eight year old boys.

Eagerly we paid close attention as our friend's spoke, some stumbling slightly over unfamiliar words. Our reading skills were yet to be developed but there were those who seemed to have a natural knack for reciting poetry. As I approached the microphone I was somewhat nervous about this new experience but was determined to speak as effectively as the best in class. Although I did have some difficulty and my lips tended to stick together. I felt that I had done a satisfactory job and confidently went back to my seat.

Eventually every student had completed his recital and Miss Woods rewound the tape from one reel to the other. As the tape was played back each student flushed with embarrassment as he heard his voice for the first time. Many had difficulty recognizing their voice and claimed that: " I don't sound like that!" There was some merriment as words were mispronounced and reading mistakes became self- evident. Grins of chagrin appeared on the faces of those with the most noticeable errors, but even they seemed to enjoy their temporary moment in the limelight.

As my turn approached and although I thought I had done reasonably well. I prepared to receive the giggles of my friends. I knew that I had read as well as some but I was totally unprepared for the contorted sounds regurgitated by the here to- fore friendly tape recorder. Smacking my lips as I sucked in air in a vain effort to speak, it was virtually impossible to recognize my pronunciation of my name. From there things went from bad to worse as I seemed to struggle with every word. The few minutes required for the other students seemed to stretch into hours as I fought to recite those simple four lines of poetry.

Just as with the other recordings my classmates started to giggle as my voice first came back from the reels of tape. Comprehending the difficulty I was experiencing as I struggled to speak, the giggles quickly turned to nervous laughter. In an attempt to stay one of the crowd I weakly joined with the laughter, an attempt that was interpreted by my fellow students as approved authorization to increase their laughter at the strange sounds coming from the front of the class. With every passing moment the laughter swelled and grew until I was drowning in a sea of ridicule. Like ocean waves, the peals of laughter slammed violently into my ears. Each blow seemed like a physical force that relentlessly drove my head down on to my desk. My weak attempt at laughter quickly turned to whimpers, then tears, then to complete despair as I lost all remaining self-esteem I felt horribly and nakedly exposed as my innocence about my speech was stripped away. My devastation was complete.

When I was able to raise my head I found that the noon hour bell had sounded and that Miss Woods and my classmates had quietly slipped away. I was relieved not to have to face them and silently slunk out of the room and made my way home for lunch. "Nothing!" was the answer I gave my mother when she asked me what was wrong; and I spent most of the noon break slowly returning to school.

Keeping my eyes downcast as I wended my way back to my desk, I would have given anything not to return to school that day. Unfortunately I had nowhere else to go and truancy was a crime of the highest order. Half of the class had returned from their lunch when I sat at my desk and all avoided my eyes as I cast furtive glances around me. My closest friend entered the room and softly approached my seat, embarrassedly blurting out "Here" he shoved a small brown paper bag filled with penny candy onto my desk. Mumbling "Thanks" I raised the hinged lid on the desk and started to put the bag of candy inside to be saved for later consumption, it took me a moment to realize that the space inside my desk was filled with other candy bags, shiny red apples, oranges and even a small tinker toy or two. In their own way my classmates had scavenged a treat for me during lunch as a "peace offering".

Yes, I was seven when I lost my innocence.

M.H. (Canada)

My Experience of Dublin Adult Stammering (DAS)

I first heard about DAS from my daughter's Speech Therapist. Initially I thought the course was for real stutterers, not for people like me who had managed to successfully hide their stutter from others. After all, to others I appeared fluent so I was okay. As my daughter's therapy progressed I began to realise that if I was to encourage her to be open and honest about her stammer then I needed to be the same about mine.

So I found myself in Balbriggan with a group who had also decided to take that step. I was apprehensive about going to the course; to openly admit to having a stammer was a huge step for me, but ultimately a huge relief. Acknowledging my stammer was an emotional experience because as a covert stammerer I had gone to such lengths to hide it from my parents, siblings, husband, children, friends and work colleagues. I learned that all my tricks such as word substitution "ems", pauses, starting sentences over etc., were just crutches I used to avoid facing up to the fact that I stammered. I also learned that covert stammerers had a lot in common with overt stammerers, in terms of how both groups feel about themselves and their speech. I found it quite difficult to stutter in front of people as hiding my stammer was so deeply embedded in my speaking that actually having someone hear and see me stutter was a terrifying prospect. I learned to use voluntary stammering to help desensitize myself to stammering and as a way of struggling less when speaking. Firstly I practiced my voluntary stammering in the safety of the group and with the therapists. The most daunting thing for me to do was to go in to the world outside and stutter, but with the help and encouragement of other participants and most of the therapists, I went into situations I would previously have avoided or avoided speaking in, such as going into the Post Office to enquire about passport express forms. I found the support of other participants really helpful as we shared experiences about how we had been affected by our stutter. I had a lot of laughs as I began to let go of some of my old crutches and see the humorous side of using them. I also shed some tears as I realized the impact a stammer had had on my life and that hiding it was not a healthy way of dealing with it.

I ended the week on a high because I would never have the same negative feelings about my stammer again but I knew that the course was only the start of me coming to terms with my speech. I also knew I could count on the ongoing support of my co-participants and the therapists. With their help I knew it was possible.

V.L. (Ireland)

Not all Christmas Presents come in wrapping paper.

I have thought long and hard before deciding to share this tale. This is a story of reaching out, albeit accidental, and of the rewards that come of doing so. To tell this kind of story seems embarrassingly boastful, but that is far from my intention. I am sharing it on the chance that it might encourage others to take a similar kind of risk. The rewards that it can bring are too great to keep to myself.

It is probably redundant to state that I stutter. Mine is a pretty mild impediment as such things go, and I have good coping skills, so most of the time it does not get in the way of my doing things. In fact I do a lot of things which most people might expect me to avoid. I dislike being embarrassed as much as anyone, but the other option is inertia which is no option. Thus it was that a few years ago, largely in response to an emergency request from the school principal in the remote fishing village where I live, that I found myself teaching elementary school art and woodshop.

I have taught on and off for years but almost entirely to adults and older teens. This was the first time I had to face children quite so young, and I had to interest them in a subject that has a pretty bad reputation for vapor – headedness among the general population. I resolved therefore to be as no nonsense, as well organized, and as thoroughly prepared as I could be. That included keeping a tight rein on my wayward tongue. I did not want to give the kids an extra excuse to devalue a wonderful, but sorely misunderstood part of their learning.

At my first meeting with the fourth grade one little redhead held herself apart from the general commotion as the class wiggled and jostled to find places at the art table for their crayons, water colors, elbows and big sheets of paper. I know too well how disorienting a noisy group can be, so I left her alone until the class was pretty well occupied with their assignment. Then I pulled up a chair next to her and asked if she wanted to draw something.

She shook her head; no. Through the whole ninety minute class she sat very still, silent and hardly moving. This scene repeated itself for several sessions. Her supervising teacher told me she was a very difficult and stubborn child and I should not worry about her being so still and quiet. It was better than when she got angry and stormed out. This teacher suggested I just let her go when, not if, she did that.

One day after I had passed out supplies and the assignment was underway, the little girl came to me. Stuttering on almost every word she asked, "Why do we have to learn to draw?" Bingo! The flash of recognition cut like a hot knife. I felt like an idiot: I had overlooked the obvious. "Why? So you can express yourself! Show people what you are thinking about." I answered, trying not to sound too intense. You of all people, I thought to myself. She blushed and turned away, but that day she began to draw.

The explosion came some weeks later in girls' woodshop class. Although most children are basically kind people, in any group there will always be some competition, teasing and formless insensitivity. I didn't see what set off the explosion. The teacher's dilemma is to keep an eye on the whole group when an individual needs some extra attention. There was a shout, a clattering of tools and wood. I looked up from the project I was helping with, to see the redhead stomping out of the woodshop in a blue fury. "What happened" I asked".

"I don't know", answered several kids. "Someone teased her I guess", said one. "She just gets mad, she does that all the time", said another. "She told me that she doesn't think she's human because she stutters and has red hair".

That hot knife again! This time it cut deep, right through the bindings which held a stampede of memories; hiding under the teacher's desk in second grade, bullies gone unanswered in the fifth, the tears of sheer frustration that did not let up until Junior High. My heart almost broke.

"Ohh, nnnooohh, that's not so!" I said - blurted really, she is every bit a human as I am. You know I stuttered to, still do. It's just oh so awfully hard when the words wont come!"

There, it was done. Two months of coping strategies, determination, tight rein and preparation; all gone in the breath of a few words, but the little girls were respectful and honestly curious. For several minutes I fielded questions, then I suggested a little role playing, that they count silently to ten before they say anything for the next few minutes. Of course the exercise soon dissolved into a mass of giggles but at the same time I could see understanding begin to take root. The children found that they were becoming impatient both with themselves and with each other.

In a town as small as this one word travels fast. The next time the art class met my redhead was visibly more relaxed. So was I, but there's more. I found myself able and even compelled to discuss the matter with my colleagues, to suggest ways to deal with the child's problems. (In case you are wondering therapy is virtually out of the question as the nearest specialist is about 450 miles away.) I dug up some un-circulated informational material from the "special education" file and circulated it. At first, to my surprise, the other teachers were far more embarrassed than I was. But in the end they were glad for the information as well as for "a view from the inside."

One day near Christmas I encountered the girl and her Grandmother in the hardware store. When the child was out of earshot for a moment the Grandmother grabbed my arm, and with a passion she said, "I want to thank you from the bottom of my heart for what you have done for my grand daughter. It has made such a difference in her life, you can't know."

Not all Christmas presents come in wrapping paper.

I am no longer teaching, I started a sign and graphics business at the end of the school year. However my redhead is one of the more or less constant stream of former students who stop to visit to watch me work and to play with my dog. She is going on twelve now, she has friends and she smiles easily. We talk together, though she still seldom speaks to adults outside of her family. Once in a while when I land in a bad block we exchange winks.

I know that if I never have an opportunity to do another unselfish thing I can rest proud of that unguarded moment, and the effect it has had on a once scared, unhappy child. It would be great if she could get the help she needs, but the world isn't always fair. What I can give her is the next best thing: the knowledge that she is not alone, and the belief that the stutter does not matter any more then she allows it to.

L.H.

A New Day.

At the age of 5
I loved mornings.
Mornings meant a start of a new day, a new life.
Another day of laughing and playing.
Being loved and encouraged
by family and pre-school teachers.
With lots of friends and people supporting me,
anxiously waiting for a new day to come.

At the age of 10.
I loved afternoons.
Afternoons meant coming home from school.
After a day of teasing and bullying, fear and humiliation,
being ridiculed and put down
by family and teachers.
With hardly any friends or support
anxiously fearing the new day to come.

At the age of 20
I loved nights.
Nights meant not to be seen, not to be heard.
Another night of crying, terrified of tomorrow.
Being totally ignored and unloved
by family and even myself.
With no friends or support what so ever
anxiously hoping for the new day never to arrive.

At the age of 30.
I once again loved mornings.
Mornings meant a new beginning, a new period of growth.
New mornings of hope and baby steps.

Trying to be myself and acknowledge my feelings.
Being accepted by family and colleagues, encouraging me on my
new path.
With new friends who stutter, support and understand
anxiously looking forward to a new day to come.
At the age of ... well... now.
I once again love tomorrow.

Afternoons mean looking back on a day of wider comfort zones
and new challenges.
New afternoons of faith in the future and in myself.
Remembering how to live, love, laugh and dream again.
Being loved, appreciated and even challenged
by family and colleagues.
With friends and support groups from all over the world
anxiously waiting for the future to come.

At the age of 50.
I want to look back at those mornings, afternoon and nights.
Mornings of being lost, afternoons of being found and nights of
being re-born.
Days full of love, life and self esteem.
To now GIVE love, life and self esteem
to family and colleagues.
And to now give support to friends all over the world,
anxiously waiting for the next generation to pass it on to.

My wish for you is
to look forward to mornings
with hope for the new day to come.
To look forward to afternoons.
and see the progress you made.
To look forward to nights

and feel good about who you are, no matter what.
With love from your family
encouragement from your colleagues
and support from your friends and fellow stutterers
anxiously waiting to help other people who stutter to believe in
themselves
and to become the beautiful person YOU are today.

Thank You.
A.S.B.

Freedom of Speech

I remember it very well, my first day in Secondary School and the teacher asking everyone to stand up and say their names. It was one of those situations that I was not able to avoid, one of those times that I wished the ground would open up and swallow me. That was the start of it, the start of five years of hell from the other students. I couldn't walk up the hallway without getting a nasty cruel comment from someone about my stammer. My stammer didn't affect me that much until Secondary School. I never answered my phone. Never went into a restaurant that was not self service and, this is a very strong word that I rarely use in my life now, but I used to hate myself. Stammering affects each individual in different ways, for me it led to me suffering from bulimia for five years in Secondary School. As ridiculous as it sounds to me now, this was my way of escaping and dealing with all of these feelings and emotions that my stammer had brought me. I was always sad, I rarely smiled and I was so unhappy within myself. I felt alone and I used to wonder what it would be like just to be able to make a phone call without stammering.

All this changed when I went on a course in November 2004. I got to experience what it felt like to be able to speak under control. Since going on this course I have achieved so many things that, in the past, I used to dream about. I have freedom in my speech. I am becoming the person that I want to be. I now love when the phone rings, I love speaking to people. I am proud of the person that I am now, and I have accepted that I have a stammer. This course has transformed my entire life; speech wise it is a transformation and in general life it has made me a stronger person. I jump at the chance of any speaking situation, and in my personal life I only surround myself with people that make me happy. It is still hard work and it may take quite a few years for me to reach eloquence, but I am happy with the way things are going now.

Eternal thanks to all the people who got me to where I am today, you all know who you are.

S.K (Ireland)

Letter received following an interview on Tipp F.M Radio

Michael,

I hope this letter finds you well. I thought I was hearing things when I heard you on the radio yesterday speaking about stammering and looking for information for your forthcoming book.

Michael, I am forty five years old and it was the first time in my life that I have heard stammering and how it affects peoples lives being discussed on local or national radio. I thought you were fantastic you know the behavior, mentality and how stammering affects the lives of people who stammer very well and you explained it very well. It was great to listen to someone who really understood what goes on in the mind of a person who stammers.

You explained the difference between an overt and a covert stammerer in a way that I had never heard before and I could really relate to everything you were saying. When I rang you after the interview your were courteous. You listened to me talk about how it felt for me every day living the life of a very covert stammerer, how it really hurts me every time that I am found out. It is seldom that I am found out because my tricks, as you so rightly called them, are second nature to me now and you explained why, which was a revelation to me.

Regarding that very negative work experience that we talked about yesterday, after hearing it, you asked if I would write it down for you to include in your book, as you thought it may help others. Yesterday I declined but I talked it over with my daughter and sister and they advised me to sleep on it. I have decided to write something for your book, you did not guarantee that it would be included and if it is not I fully understand.

About five years ago I was at work, I work in an open plan building for a large company and I am Senior Supervisor to a group of ten female employees. I have worked for this company since I left college and worked my way up to the position I now have which is Senior Control Manager. I achieved all this while all the time hiding my stuttering problem or so I thought.

One day one of the girls answered the phone in my section and she started stumbling over words as she became more flustered on the phone. When she hung up she said to two of the girls near her, "My god I sounded just like S…, there, I stuttered so much. I wonder am I catching it from her." The three girls started to giggle and I heard every word as I passed by. To describe how I felt inside at that point in time would be impossible to understand. It had such a profound affect on me that I did not return to work after lunch. I phoned in sick for the next three days, something I had never done in my entire working life.

It took me this amount of time to pick up the courage to go back to work and face my work mates. My confidence took a severe tumble; I began to communicate through memos instead of verbally it became so obvious that my Line manager took me out to lunch to see what was wrong. At first of course I denied that anything was wrong; it took two further lunches before I decided to say what had happened and how it had affected me. She was very understanding. She asked me if I realised that most of the people in my section and at Management level knew that I had a speech problem sometimes, not always only sometimes. Here I was thinking that I was so clever in hiding it so that no one knew. I was, as you called it Michael, a covert stammerer; my big secret was out. It took me a while to get used to the idea that my big secret was public knowledge, but in time I started to accept it.

Of course I still do my best to hide it from people that I meet for the first time, as I am still very sensitive to how I speak, but now I am prepared to speak about it to my family and close friends.

All the best Michael, you are a good man and just talking and listening to you has made me accept myself as a whole person. I cant wait to read your book when it comes out.

All the Best.
S.S.

Letter received following a radio interview on Roscommon Radio

Hello Michael,

Thank you for listening and for being so understanding on Thursday. You asked me to write something down to include in your book as you thought it might help other parents who may have experienced the same as me or something similar, so here goes.

My son, who is now twelve, started stammering when he was five years old. We first noticed it just after he started school and as he progressed in age it seemed to get worse and he was also very aware of how he spoke.

We brought him to Speech Therapy on four separate occasions, each session lasting about six months. His speech improved a lot while he was in a session, but as soon as he left he seemed to revert back to his stammering. When he was in school he was always very quiet even though he had lots of friends.

One day I had to collect him from school early as he had a dentist's appointment, he was eleven at the time. I arrived during the school break he was playing football in the school playground when suddenly I heard two of the boys in the group mocking how he was speaking. When I heard this it was like someone had stabbed me in the heart and twisted a sharp knife several times it was so painful.

It was quite obvious to my son how upset I was as I started to shake in the car. That situation had a profound affect on me, it also left me thinking about how my young felt if this was happening to him every day.

When we arrived home and my husband arrived home from work I told him what had happened. He became very upset as he told me he had heard our son being mocked on a few occasions but he didn't tell me as he knew I would be upset.

Our two daughters arrived home that evening, later then usual as they had basketball practice. When they walked into the kitchen they could see how upset both of us were. I asked them if they had ever heard their brother being mocked in school or while out playing. They both said they had and they both became upset.

You explained to me Michael about the emotional charge that is around a child or a person who stammers. I have experienced this first hand with my own family. I also realised that there was a huge conspiracy of silence within the family regarding our son's speech.

That evening and ever since, we talk openly to our son regarding his speech. He is more relaxed about his stammering and it has made a huge difference to him and to us as well. The conspiracy of silence is truly over.

E.W.

Letter received following a radio interview on K.C.L.R.;

Hi Michael,

It was great to hear you speak on the radio today. What you were saying made so much sense and it also gave me the strength to write this down. As I have never spoken about this before, when you mentioned the pain that stammering causes, not only to the person who stammers but maybe to a loved one as well, it really hit a cord with me.

My lovely daughter who is only five has developed a stammering problem over the past couple of months. My partner and I split up a few months ago and shortly after this she started to stammer. I think the split has had a very negative affect on her and this may be the reason she started to stammer. Maybe I am trying to convince myself that this is the reason, I don't know?

A few weeks ago as I was leaving my daughter to school she had just gotten out of the car when I heard one of her little school friends mocking how she spoke. I felt helpless, I just went numb and I didn't know what to do. I could not say a word. One of the other parents started to speak to me and I couldn't hear a word she was saying, I just nodded my head. The school bell went, I kissed and hugged my little daughter who seemed to be oblivious to what had just happened.

That day I did not go to work nor did I for the rest of the week. The pain that I felt for my little daughter was almost unbearable. Flashes of her future being mocked, bullied and all of the other negative things that I was now looking up on the Internet regarding stammering were becoming very real to me. Her pain was becoming my pain, yet she was only five years of age, surely you should not experience pain at five years of age.

I was learning that there is no cure for stammering, that more boys stammer than girls and that children grow out of it. I now pray every day that my lovely daughter will be one of the lucky ones who do.

A Mother.

Helpful Reading List

The fantastic help support and knowledge that I got from my family and friends and all the people I have met who have the same problem as myself have brought me to where I am regarding my speech today.

A very necessary part of my recovery was to get as much knowledge as I could, not only to help myself understand my speaking system but to empower and support others to achieve what I have achieved.

Any knowledge I learned I always tried my best to apply it. I found the following books a fantastic resource of information and knowledge. I would like to share my book list with you and hope it may be of benefit to you.

The Elephant and the Twig. The art of positive thinking.
Author: Geoff Thompson.
Published by Summersdale Publishers Ltd.
www.summersdale.com

Coping with Stammering.
Authors: Trudy Stewert & Jackie Turnbull.
Published by Sheldon Press.
www.sheldonpress.uk

Helping Children Cope with Stammering.
Authors: Trudy Stewert & Jackie Turnbull.

Published by Sheldon Press.
www.sheldonpress.uk

"Stammering" a Practical Guide for Teachers and other
Professionals.
Authors :   Lena Rustin
                   Francis Cook.
                   Willie Botterill.
                   Cherry Hughes.
                   Elaine Kelman
Published by David Fulton Publishers Ltd.,
www.fultonpublishers.co.uk

Understanding and Controlling Stuttering.
Author: William D. Parry Esq.
Distributed by National Stuttering Association.
www.westutter.org

The Stutterers Survival Guide.
Author: Nick Tunbridge.
Published by Addison-Wesley Publshing Company.
Also by the same author. Love Your Work and Believe in
Yourself.
www.nicktunbridge.com

How To Conquer Your Fears Of Speaking Before People.
Author: John Harrisson.
Distributed through National Stuttering Association of
America.
www.westutter.org.

Young Children Who Stutter Ages 2 to 6.
Available from National Stuttering Association.
www.westutter.org

"Bullying and Teasing" Helping Children Who Stutter.
Available from National Stuttering Assosiation.
www.westutter.org

Beyond Stammering.
Author: Dave McGuire.
Publishers Souvenir Press.
www.mcguireprogramme.com

Sometimes I Just Stutter. (Children`s Book.)
Author: Eelco de Gues.
Stuttering Foundation of America.
www.stutteringhelp.org

"Don't Pick on Me" How to Handle Bullying.
Author: Rosemary Stones.
Publishers Piccadilly Press.
Available at – www.stammering.org

Think and Grow Rich.
Author: Napoleon Hill.
Publishers Ballantine Books.
www.randomhouse.com

Master Blocking and Stuttering.
Author: Bob B. Bodenhamer.
Publishers Crown House Publishing.
www.crownhouse.co.uk

You Can if You Think You Can.
Author: Vincent Peale.
Publishers Vermilion.
www.randomhouse.co.uk

You Can Have What You Want.
Author: Michael Neill
Publishers Hay House.
www.hayhouse.co.uk

Breaking the Chain of Low Self- Esteem.
Author: Marilyn Sorensen.
Available through Amazon .com
As a Man Thinketh.
Author: James Allen
Available through Amazon.com
Feel the Fear and Do it Anyway.
Author: Susan Jeffers.
Publishers Random House.
www.randomhouse.co.uk

Speak for Yourself.
Author: John Campbell.
Publishers B.B.C Worldwide Publishing
www.bbc.co.uk

Organisations and Resources for Stuttering Information and Self-Help in Ireland

The following is a list of organisations in Ireland where you can get knowledge advice and support regarding your stammering should you ever wish to do so. This list is by no means complete as there may be some that I have not heard of. There may be other courses or devices which may be available in the marketplace which you may like to try out; if they work for you that's fantastic.

Please be aware that there is no known cure for stammering and some fraudsters do appear from time to time. They tend to have a habit of capitalising on people's desperation in finding a 'quick cure', device or method that has not been adequately tested or proven. My advice is to stick to reputable organisations. As in all things, "let the buyer beware".

Irish Stammering Association,
Carmichael House,
North Brunswick Street
Dublin 7
Telephone No. 01-8724405
www.stammeringireland.ie
e-mail. mail@stammeringireland.ie

D.A.S.
Dublin Adult Stuttering
Community Care Area 6,
Rathdown Road, Dublin
Contact: Jonathan Linklater – 01 873 0969
                          Duanna Quigley - 01-8399506
                          Noreen Murphy - 01-8825190

McGuire Programme.
www.stammering.ie
Contact: Joe O'Donnell,
                          Calhame,
                          Mountain Top,
                          Letterkenny,
                          Co. Donegal.
Telephone No. 074-9125781 Mobile No. 086-3429602.

Patmar Programme for Adults who stutter.
Contact: Maria McDonnell,
Senior Speech & Language Therapist,
Markievicz House,
Barrack Street,
Sligo.
Telephone No. 071-9155132

Patrick Kelly,
Senior Speech & Language Therapist,
Community Care Offices,
Carrick-on-Shannon,
Co. Leitrim.
Telephone No. 071-9650311

Irish Association of Speech & Language Therapist in Private
Practice. Also known as IASLTPP.
www.iasltpp.com
www.enableireland.ie
www.hearing.org/speech

Michael Palin Centre.
www.stammeringcentre.org

Sheehan Stuttering Centre.
www.stuttersc.org

European League of Stuttering Associations.
www.stuttering.ws
www.stutteringhomepage.com
www.nsastutter.org
www.stuttersfa.org

261

Worldwide Organisations and Resources for Stuttering Information and Self-Help

This list represents only a few of the organisations and other resources in operation around the world and was correct at the time of going to print.

United States.
National Stuttering Association,
119 W. 40th Street,
14th Floor,
New York,
NY 10018
USA
Newsletter; *Letting Go.*
Telephone: 1-800- WE STUTTER.
e-mail: info@WeStutter.or.
Website: www.WeStutter.org

American Speech-Language-Hearing Association,
10801 Rockville Pike,
Rockville,
MD 20852
USA
Telephone: 1-800-638-8255
Website: www.asha.org

Friends
Website: www.friendswhostutter.org

Passing Twice. GLB & T People who Stutter.
Website: www.passingtwice.com

Stuttering Foundation of America,
P.O. Box 11749
Memphis TN 38111-0749
Telephone 1-800-992-9392
Newsletter: *SFA Newsletter.*
Website: www.stuttrsfa.org

The Stuttering Home page.
Website: www.stutteringhomepage.com

Canada.

Canadian Stuttering Association,
P.O. Box 3027,
Sherwood Park, AB T8H 2TI, Canada.
Website: www.stutter.ca

Speak Easy, Inc.
95 Evergreen Avenue,
Saint John NB E2N IH4
Canada.
Website: www.speakeasycanada.com

Argentina.

Association Argentina de Tartamudez.
Website: **www.aat.org.ar**

Australia.

Australian Speak Easy Association Inc.,
Website: www.speakeasy.org.au

Austria.

Oesterreichische Selbsthilfe- Initiative Stottern.
Website: www.stotternetz.at

Belgium.

Belgium Stuttering Association.
Website: www.storreren.be

Denmark.

Foreingen for Stammere i Danmark (FSD)
Website: www.fsd.dk

France.

Association Parole-Begaiement (A.P.B.)
Website: www.begaiement.org

Germany.

Bundesvereinigung Stottererer-Selbsthilfe e V
Zulpicher Str. 58,50674, Koln Germany.
Website: www.bvss.de/

India.

Fluency Club,
C/o J.C. Nigam,
35-C Pocket I/Mayur Vihar- Phase-1
Delhi 110091, India.

International.

European League of Stuttering Associations,
Website: www.stuttering.ws
(see website for list of member organisations)

International Fluency Association.
Website: www.theifa.org

International Stuttering Association
Website: www.stutterisa.org
(see website for list of member organisations)

Israel.

AMBI – Israeli Stuttering Association
Website: www.ambi.org.il *(in Hebrew)*

Japan.

Japan Stuttering Project
Shinji Ito c/o Kazue Shinji,
17-3 Monamiogi-cho Kamigamo
Kita- Ku, Kyoto 603, Japan.

The Netherlands.

Nederlands Stottervereniging "Demosthenes"
Post Box 119, NL- 3500 AC Utrect, Netherlands.
Website: www.stotteren.nl

New Zealand.

New Zealand Speak Easy Association, Inc.
P.O Box 16554,
Hornby, Christchurch, New Zealand.
Website: www.shopzone.co.nz/speakeasy

Norway.
NIFS.
Postbox 4568, Nydalen 0404, Oslo, Norway.
Website: www.stamming.no

South Africa.
Speak Easy Stuttering Association.
Website: www.speakeasy.org.za

Sweden.
SSR.- Swedish Stuttering Association,
P.O.Box 1386,
172 27 Sundbyberg, Sweden
Website: www.stamning.se

United Kingdom.
The British Stammering Association,
15, Old Ford Road, London E2 9PJ, England
Newsletter: *Speaking Out*
Website: www.stammering.org